Core Conditions for Medical and Surgical Finals

Core Conditions for Medical and Surgical Finals

Kristen Davies, MBChB (Honours), MRes (Distinction)
Academic Foundation Doctor
Northumbria Healthcare NHS Foundation Trust
Training Fellow
Newcastle University
UK

Editorial Advisor
Shadaba Ahmed, FRCS, FRCS-ORL/HNS, DLO, MoAME, MCPS, FCPS
ENT Consultant and Lead HN Services
University Hospitals of Morecombe Bay NHS Foundation Trust
Honorary Lecturer, Lancaster University
Honorary Teacher, Liverpool University
UK

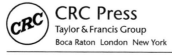
CRC Press
Taylor & Francis Group
Boca Raton London New York

CRC Press is an imprint of the
Taylor & Francis Group, an **informa** business

First edition published 2021
by CRC Press
6000 Broken Sound Parkway NW, Suite 300, Boca Raton, FL 33487-2742

and by CRC Press
2 Park Square, Milton Park, Abingdon, Oxon, OX14 4RN

© 2021 Taylor & Francis Group, LLC

CRC Press is an imprint of Taylor & Francis Group, LLC

ISBN: 9781138331181 (hbk)
ISBN: 9781138331037 (pbk)
ISBN: 9780429447433 (ebk)

Typeset in Frutiger
by Nova Techset Private Limited, Bengaluru & Chennai, India

CONTENTS

PREFACE

Core Conditions for Medical and Surgical Finals is a book primarily designed to aid medical students in preparation for their final examinations at medical school. These examinations are usually the last formal assessments prior to beginning life as a junior doctor. Even uttering the 'F' word (finals, that is) can strike shivers down the spine of medical students up and down the country. As such, I have drawn upon my experience of sitting my medical school finals and the notes I made to create *Core Conditions* in an effort to try and make your revision an easier (and hopefully stress-free!) process.

Finals are ultimately a test of clinical competence and confidence to ensure that you are going to be a safe doctor. You don't need to know the ins and outs of Waldenstrom's macroglobulinemia (don't worry, I had to Google it too) but you do need to show that you can recognise and manage common medical presentations. As the age-old saying goes, 'common things are common'. If you know the core conditions inside out, then you have a good platform for succeeding in your finals. That's where *Core Conditions* comes in. We hope that this book will provide you with the core knowledge to use as a platform for your final examinations.

Best of luck in your examinations!

Dr Kristen Davies
Academic Foundation Doctor

ACKNOWLEDGEMENTS

To Mum and Dad, for giving me the all of the encouragement and support I could ask for. Thank you!

To Sophie, for giving me the motivation to get this project over the line. You are *the* best.

To Lancaster Medical School, for giving me a chance when no one else did.

AUTHOR

Kristen Davies, MBChB (Honours), MRes (Distinction), is currently an academic FY2 doctor in the North East of England. He read medicine at Lancaster Medical School, graduating with honours with distinction in 2018. He was awarded the Chancellor's Medal for outstanding academic achievement during his studies. Kristen additionally holds an intercalated Masters of Research (MRes) in Medical Sciences from Newcastle University. He is currently pursuing a career in academic rheumatology and medical education and has been awarded a British Education Award in 2019 for his efforts.

CONTRIBUTORS

Shadaba Ahmed, FRCS-ORL/HNS, DLO, MoAME, MCPS, FCPS
Consultant ENT Surgeon
University Hospitals of Morecambe Bay
Lancaster, UK

Ela Akay, MBBS, MRCP
Consultant Neurologist
Newcastle upon Tyne Hospitals
Newcastle upon Tyne, UK

Adrian Brodison, MBChB, FRCP
Consultant Cardiologist and Clinical Lead for
  Cardiology
University Hospitals of Morecambe Bay
Lancaster, UK

Marwan Bukhari, MBBS, PhD, FRCP
Consultant Rheumatologist
University Hospitals of Morecambe Bay
Lancaster, UK

Ian Chadwick, MD, FRCP
Consultant Physician
University Hospitals of Morecambe Bay
Lancaster, UK

Colin Cutting, MBBS, FRCS
Consultant Urologist
University Hospitals of Morecambe Bay
Lancaster, UK

Mark Garside, BMedSci, MBBS, MD, MRCP
Consultant Stroke Physician
Northumbria Healthcare NHS Foundation Trust
Northumberland, UK

David Howarth, MBChB, FRCP
Consultant Haematologist
University Hospitals of Morecambe Bay
Lancaster, UK

Rachel Isba, BM, BCh, MA, MPH, PhD, FFPH, FAcadMEd
Consultant in Paediatric Emergency Medicine and
  Public Health
Associate Dean for Engagement for the Faculty of
  Health and Medicine
North Manchester General Hospital
Manchester, UK

Joanne John, MBChB, DFSRH, PGCert (Med.Ed), MRCP, Dip.GUM, LFFLM
Specialty Registrar Genitourinary Medicine and
  HIV/Forensic Medical Examiner
University Hospitals of Morecambe Bay
Lancaster, UK

Svetlana Kavaklieva-Shtarbanova, MBBS, MRCP
Consultant Dermatologist
University Hospitals of Morecambe Bay
Lancaster, UK

Paul Marshall, MBBS, FRCS (Ortho)
Consultant Orthopaedic and Trauma Surgeon
University Hospitals of Morecambe Bay
Lancaster, UK

Sally Marshall, MBChB, MD, FRCP
Professor of Diabetes and Honorary Consultant
  Physician
Newcastle upon Tyne Hospitals NHS Foundation Trust
Newcastle upon Tyne, UK

Jonathan Miller, MBBS, MRCP
Consultant Respiratory Physician
Northumbria Healthcare NHS Foundation Trust
Northumberland, UK

John Nixon, MD, FRCP
Consultant Neurologist
University Hospitals of Morecambe Bay
Lancaster, UK

Rikesh Patel, BSc, MBChB, MRCP
Specialist Registrar in Rheumatology and General
 Internal Medicine
Salford Royal NHS Foundation Trust
Manchester, UK

Rhys H Thomas, BSc, MBChB, MRCP, MSc, PhD
Intermediate Clinical Fellow and Honorary Consultant
 in Epilepsy
Newcastle upon Tyne Hospitals
Newcastle upon Tyne, UK

Paul Wilson, MBChB, FRCSEd, FRCS (Gen)
Consultant General Surgeon
University Hospitals of Morecambe Bay
Lancaster, UK

Cardiology

1.1 ACUTE CORONARY SYNDROME (ACS)

DEFINITION

A group of conditions with a common underlying pathology: plaque formation, thrombosis and inflammation.

The usual cause is an atheromatous plaque rupturing a coronary artery, which either fully/partially obstructs.

Differentiation between the conditions is determined by the presence of (1) cardiac sounding chest pain (chest pain in the chest/jaw/back with nausea/sweating for >15 minutes), (2) troponin rise, (3) ST-segment elevation.

Unstable Angina (UA) – frequent cardiac chest pain, often at rest, **without** troponin rise. ECG changes such as ST depression or T wave inversion may or may not be present but are often transient.

Non-ST-Elevation Myocardial Infarction (NSTEMI) – cardiac chest pain **with** troponin rise **without** ST elevation.

ST-Elevation Myocardial Infarction – cardiac chest pain **AND** troponin rise **AND** ST-elevation ECG changes.

EPIDEMIOLOGY

Ischaemic heart disease (IHD) is the most common cause of death in the UK.

Modifiable risk factors: Hypertension, smoking, ↑ cholesterol, type 2 diabetes mellitus, obesity, sedentary lifestyle.

Non-modifiable risk factors: Family history, increasing age, sex (M > F until menopause when M = F).

AETIOLOGY/PATHOLOGY

The inflammatory process of atherosclerosis of the coronary arteries occurs over time, resulting in the development of a plaque. Symptoms of ACS occur when there is rupture of the plaque, resulting in platelet activation, thrombosis formation and occlusion.

CLINICAL PRESENTATION

Most common symptoms include central crushing chest pain, which may radiate to the jaw/arm with an associated sympathetic response (nausea, vomiting, sweating). Individuals with diabetes may have a 'silent MI' without chest pain.

Timing of the chest pain, and the timing of blood taking, is important for interpretation of troponin blood tests.

EXAMINATION

Signs include: AF (IHD is a major cause), hypertension, signs of ↑ cholesterol (arcus lipidus, xanthalasma), surgical scars (median sternotomy + venous graft harvest scars on lower limbs → previous CABG).

INVESTIGATIONS

Bedside: Serial ECGs (detect ECG changes – see box), BM.

- Bloods: Troponin (myocardial injury), FBC (anaemia – can lead to a Type 2 MI), glucose, lipids, U&Es (↓ K^+ – arrhythmogenic).
- Imaging: CXR (exclude other causes of acute chest pain), echocardiogram (check cardiac size and function).

DIFFERENTIAL DIAGNOSIS

Acute chest pain differentials include: Cardiac causes (angina, pericarditis, aortic dissection, heart failure), respiratory causes (pneumothorax, pneumonia, pulmonary embolism), trauma, musculoskeletal, gastrooesophageal reflux disease, costochondritis and anxiety.

STEMI ECG changes

- Hyperacute T waves
- ST elevation
- Inverted T waves
- Pathological Q waves

Type 2 MI

- MI secondary to ischaemia due to either increased O_2 demand or decreased O_2 supply

Absolute contraindications to fibrinolysis

- Previous haemorrhagic stroke
- Stroke <6 months
- Active internal bleeding
- Aortic dissection

MANAGEMENT

Acute management

Prehospital management: **M²ONA**: **M**orphine, **M**etoclopramide, **O**xygen (if saturations <94%), **N**itrates, **A**spirin 300 mg

If *STEMI*: If **primary percutaneous coronary intervention** (**PCI**) can be delivered <120 minutes from the onset of chest pain → give a second antiplatelet (ticagrelor/clopidogrel) and LMWH prior to PCI.

If PCI cannot be delivered <120 minutes → give fibrinolysis (alteplase or tenecteplase). It is usual to transfer for PCI following thrombolysis 'drip and ship' model if revascularisation does not occur.

If *NSTEMI/UA*: Give **antiplatelets** (aspirin and clopidogrel/ ticagrelor) + **antithrombin** therapy (fondaparinux or LMWH unless patient has a high risk of bleeding). A risk score will often be applied (e.g. TIMI/HEART/GRACE). If a patient scores highly enough, a transfer for angiography within 96 h is recommended.

Chronic disease management
Non-pharmacological
- Education about the disease
- Offer a cardiac rehabilitation programme
- Address modifiable factors: Stop smoking, healthy diet, physical activity, lose weight if overweight, alcohol consumption within recommended limits
- Driving: Car/motorcycle – stop driving for 1 month; bus/HGV driver – inform DVLA
- Sexual activity can be resumed when comfortable to do so, usually 4 weeks after MI

Pharmacological
Table 1.1.1 presents the drugs used in the treatment of ACS.

Secondary prevention medications (**5 As**) – unless there is an allergy
- **A**spirin
- Another **A**ntiplatelet for 12 months (e.g. ticagrelor/clopidogrel)
- **A**CE inhibitor
- **A**tenolol (a beta-blocker)
- **A**torvastatin (high-dose statin)

Surgical
Coronary artery bypass graft (CABG) can be considered for a stable patient at intermediate/higher risk of adverse cardiovascular events, although usually only for those who are unsuitable for PCI or with coronary anatomy suggesting better outcome with surgery.

COMPLICATIONS POST-STEMI
- Ischaemic: Angina, re-infarction
- Mechanical: Heart failure, mitral valve dysfunction, ventricular wall rupture (leads to tamponade)

Table 1.1.1 Common drugs used in the treatment of ACS

Medication	Mechanism of action
Aspirin	Blocks thromboxane A2 production
Clopidogrel/Ticagrelor/Prasugrel	Block P2Y12 receptor, preventing platelet aggregation
Fondaparinux	Activates antithrombin III, which inhibits factor Xa
Bivalirudin	Reversible direct thrombin inhibitor
Alteplase	Tissue plasminogen activator
Eptifibatide/Tirofiban	Glycoprotein IIb/IIIa inhibitors

- Arrhythmic: Complete heart block (particularly if the right coronary artery is affected as this usually supplies the AV node)
- Embolic: Stroke/peripheral clot
- Inflammatory: Early pericarditis, Dressler syndrome (2–6 weeks post-MI)

TYPES OF STEMI AND TERRITORIES AFFECTED
- Anterior: Usually affects the left anterior descending (LAD) – ST elevation in leads V2–V5
- Inferior: Usually affects the right coronary artery – ST elevation in leads II, III, aVF
- Lateral: Usually affects the left circumflex artery – ST elevation in leads I and aVL
- Posterior: Usually affects the right coronary artery – ST depression in V1–V3
- Septal: Usually affects the septal branches – ST elevation in V3–V4
- Anterolateral: Usually affects the LAD – ST elevation in V4–V6, I and aVL

1.2 HEART FAILURE

DEFINITION

Heart failure is an inability of the heart to maintain sufficient cardiac output, as a result of structural or functional impairment of ventricular filling or ejection, to meet demand.

EPIDEMIOLOGY

Around 900,000 people in the UK have heart failure and incidence and prevalence increase steeply with age.

Average age of diagnosis is 76 years.

AETIOLOGY

Heart failure is the final common pathway of heart disease. It can be caused by any condition that affects one of following:

- **Myocardium**: Ischaemic heart disease, cardiomyopathy, cardiac tamponade, arrhythmias
- **Valvular dysfunction**: Stenosis or regurgitation of the mitral/aortic/tricuspid/pulmonary valve
- **Outflow obstruction**: Hypertension (systemic + pulmonary), aortic stenosis, coarctation of the aorta

High-output heart failure is considered separately and can be caused by anaemia, thyrotoxicosis and Paget disease.

PATHOLOGY

The pathophysiology of heart failure can be described by Starling's Law: as the preload (end-diastolic volume) increases due to the initial dysfunction of the myocardium, contractility increases to maintain ejection fraction (EF). As preloads increase, however, contractility cannot maintain EF beyond a certain point, and the EF decreases. Cardiac output is then maintained by increasing total peripheral resistance and heart rate, which both contribute further to heart failure. These mechanisms contribute towards the following problems:

- **Activation of the renin–angiotensin–aldosterone system** (due to ↓ CO) → worsening **hypertension**
- **Myocardial remodelling**: Initially myocyte hypertrophy to maintain contractility (**LVH**). As fluid retention increases, the myocardium dilates to make room for this fluid, resulting in a displaced apex
- Release of **brain natriuretic peptide** (**BNP**) in response to stretching of the myocardium, which can be measured in the **serum**

CLINICAL PRESENTATION

- Breathlessness that may occur on exertion, at rest, lying flat (orthopnoea), nocturnal cough or waking from sleep gasping for breath (paroxysmal nocturnal dyspnoea). Patients may also produce white/pink frothy sputum

Table 1.2.1 Left- vs. right-sided heart failure

Left-sided heart failure (pulmonary congestion)	Right-sided heart failure (systemic congestion)
Fine bi-basal crepitations (pulmonary oedema)	↑JVP
Displaced apex beat (displaced to mid-axillary line)	Reduced air entry and stony dull percussion note (transudative pleural effusion)
Gallop rhythm (S3 – indicates a volume overload in the ventricle)	Peripheral oedema
	Hepatomegaly
JVP often elevated due to back pressure on the right heart	Ascites

- Fluid retention (ankle swelling, feeling bloated, weight gain)
- Other symptoms may include fatigue or reduced exercise tolerance, or loss of consciousness/syncope

EXAMINATION

Findings on examination can be split anatomically into left- and right-sided heart failure (congestive if coexist) (*Table 1.2.1*).

General signs to examine for include raised BP, cyanosis, tachyopnoea and tachycardia.

INVESTIGATIONS

- Bedside: ECG (looking for evidence of LVH – voltage criteria see box).
- Bloods: FBC (anaemia), U&Es (checking for evidence of AKI/CKD), ABG, BNP, TFTs (hyperthyroidism), LFTs.
- Imaging: CXR, echocardiogram.

DIFFERENTIAL DIAGNOSIS

For breathlessness: COPD, asthma, pneumonia, PE, lung cancer, anxiety, fibrosis, pneumothorax.

For peripheral oedema: Dependent oedema (venous insufficiency), nephrotic syndrome, drugs (amlodipine, NSAIDs), hypoalbuminaema (renal/hepatic failure).

MANAGEMENT
Acute pulmonary oedema

Management for acute pulmonary oedema can be remembered with the mnemonic **IPODMAN**: Intravenous access, Position (sit the patient upright), Oxygen (high flow), Diuretic (IV furosemide – to remove fluid from the lungs), Morphine (helps to ease breathlessness), Antiemetic (given with morphine to reduce opioid-induced nausea), **N**itrates (infusion of isosorbide mononitrate).

Continuous Positive Airway Pressure (CPAP) can be given to help improve oxygenation if medical treatments fail.

Consider **cause-specific treatment** for acute pulmonary oedema:

- MI/ischaemia: **PCI/thrombolysis**
- Bradycardia: **Temporary pacing**
- Tachyarrhythmia: **Amiodarone/DC cardioversion**
- Anaemia: **Blood transfusion with furosemide**

Chronic disease management

Non-pharmacological

- Education about the condition: Advise the patient about reporting worsening symptoms of heart failure
- Monitor weight at home to detect fluid retention or worsening heart failure
- Dietary advice: Avoid excessive salt intake and if symptomatic they should restrict fluid intake
- Smoking cessation and reduce alcohol consumption if above normal limits
- Exercise; Regular low-intensity physical activity

Pharmacological

- NICE Guidelines 2010 state:
  - *First-line treatment* for all patients is an **ACE-inhibitor + β-blocker and often spironolactone or eplerenone**
  - *Second-line treatment* is either an **angiotensin II receptor blocker** if ACE intolerant or **hydralazine** in combination with a **nitrate if ACE or ARB causes acute renal dysfunction**
  - *Third line treatment* should be considered if symptoms persist with either cardiac resynchronisation therapy, digoxin or ivabradine
- Loop diuretics should be given for fluid overload
- Offer annual influenza vaccine and a one-off pneumococcal vaccine
- If a patient has cardiovascular risk factors, then they may need treatment with an antiplatelet and a statin

The following drugs have been shown to reduce mortality in chronic heart failure:

- ACE inhibitors
- Spironolactone
- Beta-blockers
- Hydralazine with nitrates
- Recently, ivabradine in tachycardic patients
- Sacubitril/valsartan

Chest x-ray findings in acute pulmonary oedema

ABCDE

- **A**lveolar shadowing (bat-wings sign)
- **B** lines (interstitial oedema)
- **C**ardiomegaly
- **D**iversion of blood to upper lobe
- **E**ffusion

Voltage criteria for diagnosing LVH

Limb leads

- R wave in lead I + S wave in lead III >35 mm
- R wave in aVL >11 mm
- R wave in aVF >20 mm
- S wave in aVR >14 mm

Precordial leads

- R wave in V4, V5 or V6 >26 mm
- R wave in V5 or V6 plus S wave in V1 >35 mm
- Largest R wave plus largest S wave in precordial leads >45 mm

---

REFERENCE

National Institute for Health and Care Excellence. Chronic heart failure. https://www.nice.org.uk/guidance/ng106

1.3 HYPERTENSION

DEFINITION

Hypertension is defined as a persistently raised arterial blood pressure (BP). It should be suspected if systolic BP is sustained above 140 mmHg or diastolic BP is sustained above 90 mmHg.

EPIDEMIOLOGY

Hypertension is common and increases with age. Risk factors include increasing age, sex (M>F), lack of physical activity, stress, high salt diet, obesity and ethnicity.

AETIOLOGY

Primary or essential hypertension (90%) has no identifiable cause.

Secondary hypertension (10%) can be caused by **renal** problems (renal artery stenosis, glomerulonephritis, diabetic nephropathy, polycystic kidney disease), **endocrine** problems (phaeochromocytoma, Cushing syndrome, Conn syndrome, congenital adrenal hyperplasia, acromegaly), **drugs** (oral contraceptive pill, steroids, MAO inhibitors) and **pregnancy** (preeclampsia).

PATHOLOGY

The pathogenesis of hypertension is unclear. Chronically elevated BP leads to structural vessel wall changes that increase the thickness of the wall, which reduces the diameter of the lumen. This increased mechanical stress promotes atherosclerosis. The increase in total peripheral resistance (afterload) leads to left ventricular hypertrophy. As a memory aid, the changes involved in hypertension can cause microvascular and macrovascular complications.

Macrovascular complications

- Stroke
- Peripheral vascular disease
- Ischaemic heart disease

Microvascular complications

- Chronic kidney disease
- Hypertensive retinopathy
- Peripheral neuropathy (more likely with concurrent diabetes)

CLINICAL PRESENTATION

Hypertension is often an incidental finding on examination. If undiagnosed and untreated for a period of time, patients may present with complications relating to end-organ damage.

EXAMINATION

When examining a patient with hypertension you need to look for evidence of the cause and for the presence of complications of hypertension.

Examination should include:

- Full cardiovascular assessment (including blood pressure, apex position and peripheral vascular examination)
- Auscultation of the lung bases for evidence of pulmonary oedema
- Abdominal examination looking for enlarged kidneys, renal bruits and an abdominal aortic aneurysm
- Ophthalmoscopy checking for end-organ damage

INVESTIGATIONS

- Bedside: BP, ECG (LVH), ophthalmoscopy (retinopathy), urinalysis (nephropathy), urinary catecholamines (phaeochromocytoma).
- Bloods: FBC, U&Es, lipid profile, blood glucose, serum renin:aldosterone ratio (Conn syndrome).
- Imaging: CXR/echocardiogram (heart failure), angiography (renal artery stenosis).

If a patient's BP is found to be >140/90, NICE recommends taking a second measurement and confirming a diagnosis of hypertension with **ambulatory blood pressure monitoring** (**ABPM**).

Grading of hypertension (NICE Guidelines)

Stage 1 hypertension: Clinic BP at least 140/90 mmHg, and subsequent ABPM daytime average or HBPM average at least 135/85 mmHg

Stage 2 hypertension: Clinic BP at least 160/100 mmHg, and subsequent ABPM daytime average or HBPM average at least 150/95 mmHg

Severe hypertension: Clinic systolic BP at least 180 mmHg or clinic diastolic BP at least 110 mmHg

Accelerated hypertension: Clinic BP usually higher than 180/110 mmHg with signs of papilloedema and/or retinal haemorrhage or other evidence of acute and progressive end-organ damage

---

Chronic disease management
Non-pharmacological

- Education about the condition and why it is important to treat (e.g. to reduce risk of stroke/IHD)

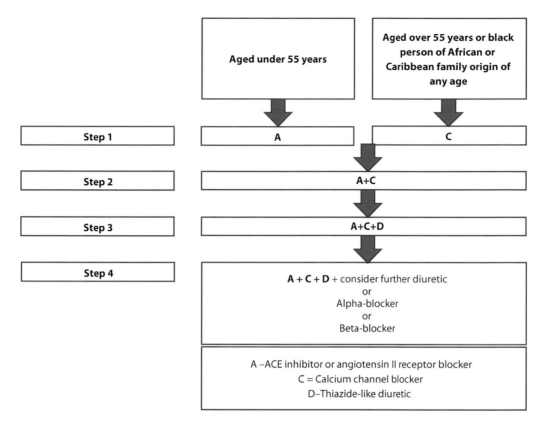

Figure 1.3.1 NICE hypertension management algorithm.

- Assess cardiovascular risk using a **QRISK2 score**
- Offer lifestyle advice on diet and exercise, stress management, smoking and alcohol consumption
- Carry out tests for end-organ damage and secondary causes of hypertension (if not already done)
- Inform patients of **annual testing** for BP and end-organ damage

Pharmacological

- Offer treatment for stage 1 hypertension if there is evidence of end-organ damage, diabetes, renal disease, cardiovascular disease or a QRISK2 score >20% using a stepwise algorithm (Figure 1.3.1)
- For treatment of stage 2 hypertension, NICE recommends following a stepwise algorithm (Figure 1.3.1)
- Prescribe antiplatelet and statin therapy for patients with a QRISK2 score >10%

REFERENCE

National Institute for Health and Care Excellence. Hypertension in adults: diagnosis and management. https://www.nice.org.uk/guidance/cg127

1.4 VALVULAR HEART DISEASE

When examining a murmur, always time the auscultation of the murmur with simultaneous carotid palpation. During systole, you will feel the pulse; during diastole, the murmur is heard after or before the pulse.

AORTIC STENOSIS

This is the most common heart murmur and presents as an **ejection systolic murmur** heard over the second right intercostal space, which **radiates to the carotids** (Figure 1.4.1). Best heard sitting forwards and breathing out.

- Causes: (1) Degenerative calcification (>65 years), (2) bicuspid valve (<65 years), (3) rheumatic heart disease.
- Can also occur as supravalvular (Williams syndrome) or subvavular (HOCM and subvalvular membranes).
- Symptoms: Memory aid: **SAD** as patients may have exertional **S**yncope, **A**ngina and **D**yspnoea.
- O/E: Ejection systolic murmur (heard loudest over the second R intercostal space and radiates to the carotids), narrow pulse pressure, left ventricular hypertrophy.
- Investigations: ECG (LVH, LAD, AV-block), CXR (calcified aortic valve of limited value, LVH), echocardiogram (diagnostic).
- Management: Observe if asymptomatic; if symptomatic then consider a valve replacement.

> **Note**: Aortic *sclerosis* (a term no longer used: either AV thickening or very mild AS) is senile degeneration of the aortic valve where there is an ejection systolic murmur without carotid radiation and a normal pulse.

AORTIC REGURGITATION

Presents as an **early diastolic murmur** with various other clinical features (Figure 1.4.2).

> **Tip**: All diastolic murmurs are soft. If you can hear a loud murmur it **is not** diastolic.

Causes: (1) Valve disease (rheumatic heart disease, endocarditis, CTD, bicuspid valve) or aortic root disease (dissection, spondyloarthropathies [ankylosing spondylitis], hypertension, collagen problems [Marfan syndrome]).

- Symptoms: Exertional dyspnoea, orthopnoea, paroxysmal nocturnal dyspnoea, angina, syncope, CCF.
- O/E: Early diastolic murmur best heard down left sternal edge, exacerbated by sitting forwards and breathing out, wide pulse pressure, collapsing pulse, displaced apex (due to fluid overload).

Eponymous signs
- Quincke: Pulsating capillaries in nail beds.
- Corrigan/water hammer: Collapsing pulse.
- De Musset: Nodding head with heartbeat.
- Durosier: Diastolic murmur over femoral artery generated from femoral artery compression.
- Austin Flint: Mid-diastolic murmur in severe AR from partial closure of anterior mitral cusps.
- Traube: Pistol-shot femorals.
- Investigations: ECG (LVH), CXR (cardiomegaly, pulmonary oedema), echocardiogram (diagnostic).
- Management: Reduce systolic hypertension (ACE-inhibitors). Surgery if increasing symptoms.

Mitral regurgitation

Presents as a pan-systolic murmur heard at the apex of the heart radiating to the axilla (Figure 1.4.3). Best heard rolling onto left-hand side and breathing out.

- Causes: (1) Papillary muscle dysfunction/chordal rupture (post-MI), (2) dilated cardiomyopathy, (3) rheumatic fever/IE, (4) CTD.
- Symptoms: Dyspnoea, palpitations, fatigue.
- O/E: Pan-systolic murmur heard at the 5th intercostal space, mid-clavicular apex of the heart radiating to the axilla. AF, displaced thrusting apex (fluid overload), soft S1, LVF (S3, pulmonary oedema), loud P2 and right ventricular heave (pulmonary hypertension).
- Investigations: ECG (LVH, AF ± p-mitrale), CXR (pulmonary oedema, cardiomegaly), echocardiogram.
- Management: Control rate if in AF and anticoagulated. Diuretics for fluid overload. Surgery for deteriorating symptoms.

Mitral stenosis

Presents as a mid-diastolic murmur best heard on rolling to left-hand side and breathing out (Figure 1.4.4).

Also exacerbated by activity, e.g. raising legs a few times off the bed, with an opening snap and tapping apex beat. Loudest at the apex.

- Causes: (1) Rheumatic fever, (2) congenital.
- Symptoms: Palpitations, dyspnoea, fatigue, haemoptysis (from pulmonary hypertension), chest pain.
- O/E: Malar flush (CO_2 retention), mid-diastolic murmur, opening snap, tapping apex beat (not displaced). A Graham-Steell murmur may occur (high-pitched early diastolic murmur heard at left sternal edge. Caused by pulmonary regurgitation secondary to mitral stenosis). JVP may be raised.

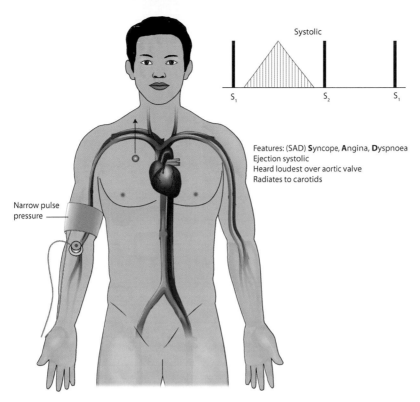

Systolic

Features: (SAD) **S**yncope, **A**ngina, **D**yspnoea
Ejection systolic
Heard loudest over aortic valve
Radiates to carotids

Narrow pulse pressure

Figure 1.4.1 Aortic stenosis.

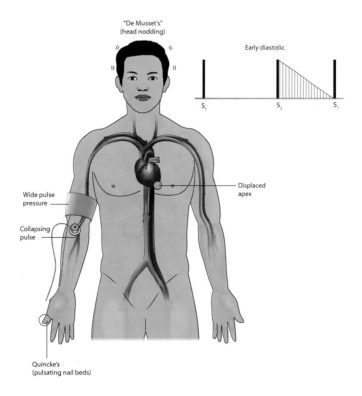

"De Musset's" (head nodding)

Early diastolic

Wide pulse pressure

Collapsing pulse

Displaced apex

Quincke's (pulsating nail beds)

Figure 1.4.2 Aortic regurgitation.

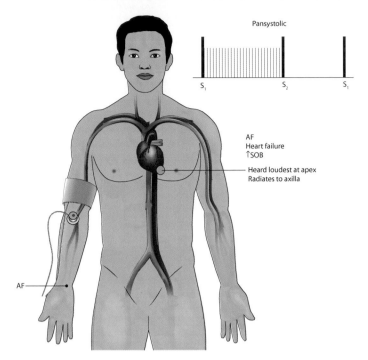

Figure 1.4.3 Mitral regurgitation.

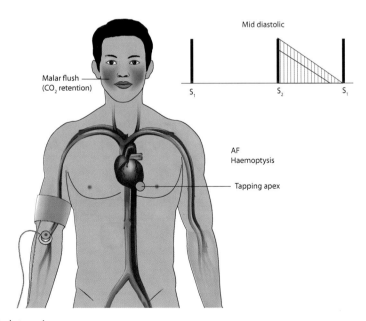

Figure 1.4.4 Mitral stenosis.

- Investigations: ECG (AF, p-mitrale, RVH, RAD), CXR (left atrial enlargement, pulmonary oedema), echocardiogram (diastolic).

- Management: In AF rate control + anticoagulation. Diuretics to reduce fluid and preload. Surgery (balloon valvuloplasty or valve replacement).

1.5 INFECTIVE ENDOCARDITIS

DEFINITION
Infective endocarditis (IE) is an infection that affects the endocardium of the heart, leading to local valvular problems and systemic problems, such as septicaemia and immunological deposition.

EPIDEMIOLOGY
IE occurs worldwide and is more common among IVDUs, immunosuppressed patients and those with prosthetic heart valves.

AETIOLOGY
IE can be caused by a variety of organisms, which usually enter the circulation through the skin to cause bacteraemia:

- *Staphylococcus aureus* (common in IVDUs and thus right-sided heart valves as entering through venous circulation)
- *Streptococcus viridans*
- Coagulase negative staphylococci (*S. epidermidis*) (associated with prosthetic valves)
- *Streptococcus bovis* (associated with colorectal cancer)
- Rarely, HACEK bacteria (see box)
- Non-infective endocarditis (SLE – Liebman-Sachs), malignancy

---

HACEK organisms

- *H*aemophilus spp.
- *A*ctinobacillus spp.
- *C*ardiobacterium spp.
- *E*ikenella corrodens
- *K*ingella spp.

PATHOLOGY
IE develops on the valvular endocardium which has developed endothelial damage due to blood flow. Platelets and fibrin adhere to the surface and create an environment where bacteria can colonise the thrombus and form a vegetation.

CLINICAL PRESENTATION
IE classically presents with either an acute or subacute course. The crux of the clinical presentation is fever, heart murmur (although this does not have to be present) and septicaemia.

Acute course: Presents with acute heart failure ± emboli (e.g. septic emboli) with a new murmur and fever. Fifty percent occur on otherwise healthy valves.

Subacute course: Tends to affect previously abnormal valves. Patients will initially complain of vague symptoms with worsening heart failure over weeks to months.

The inflammatory nature of IE leads to immune complex deposition and may cause a vasculitis affecting the kidney (haematuria/glomerulonephritis) and the eye (Roth spots – retinal haemorrhage). Immune complexes may be deposited in the hands, and these are termed either Osler nodes (painful lesions on distal fingers) or Janeway lesions (painless lesions on palms). In subacute IE, splenomegaly may occur.

The important thing to remember is that **fever + a new murmur = IE** until proven otherwise.

EXAMINATION
- Hands: Look for clubbing, splinter haemorrhages, presence of Osler nodes or Janeway lesions
- Examine for the presence of a tachycardia (septic)
- Arms: Measure BP (may be hypotensive if septic)
- Face: Perform ophthalmoscopy looking for Roth spots
- Perform a cardiovascular examination looking for a murmur
- Perform an abdominal examination looking for splenomegaly
- Dipstick the patient's urine looking for the presence of haematuria

INVESTIGATIONS
- Bedside: BP (sepsis), urine dipstick (haematuria), ECG (long PR interval if aortic root abscess).
- Bloods: FBC (infection), U&Es (renal involvement), blood cultures (sepsis + for Duke criteria – see Diagnosis), inflammatory markers (↑ ESR/CRP), lactate (sepsis).
- Imaging: CXR (cardiomegaly), echocardiogram (needed for Duke criteria).

DIAGNOSIS
The Duke criteria are used to diagnose IE. The tool is divisible into major and minor criteria.

Major criteria
- **Positive blood cultures** (typical organisms on two separate occasions or persistent bacteraemia from at least two blood cultures taken >12 hours apart).
- **Endocardium involvement** (positive echocardiogram showing a vegetation or abscess, or a new valvular regurgitation or direct histological or microbiological confirmation from a pathological specimen.)

Minor criteria
- Predisposing heart condition or IVDU
- Fever >38°C

11

- Positive blood cultures that do not meet major criteria
- Vascular/immunological phenomena: Osler nodes, Janeway lesions, clubbing, splinter haemorrhages, Roth spots, petechiae or purpura
- Positive echocardiogram that does not meet major criteria

Infective endocarditis is diagnosed by:

- Two major criteria, or
- One major criterion and three minor criteria, or
- Five minor criteria

MANAGEMENT

Management of IE involves giving initial empirical antibiotics followed by switching once the organism is identified. If patients are in acute heart failure or septic, this needs to be managed acutely. Serial blood cultures can be taken within the first few hours if patient is unwell and do not have to wait 12 hours.

Early discussion with a consultant microbiologist is recommended.

Pharmacological

Empirical antibiotic therapy involves using a penicillin, such as amoxicillin or benzylpenicillin (unless allergic)

Table 1.5.1 Examples of specific therapies for organisms grown in infective endocarditis

Organism	Therapy
Staphylococci	Flucloxacillin
Prosthetic valve and staphylococci	Flucloxacillin + rifampicin + gentamicin
Streptococci	Benzylpenicillin + gentamicin

with gentamicin (*Table 1.5.1*). Antibiotic therapy often needs to be continued for prolonged periods of time (e.g. 6 weeks).

Surgical

Surgical interventions may be indicated if there is:

- Severe valvular malfunction
- Presence of an aortic abscess
- Infections resistant to antibiotics
- Recurrent emboli after antibiotic therapy
- A very large vegetation

1.6 ATRIAL FIBRILLATION

DEFINITION
Atrial fibrillation (AF) is a common arrhythmia that results from irregular, disorganised atrial contraction leading to an irregular ventricular rhythm. AF can be classified as either paroxysmal, persistent or permanent.

Paroxysmal	Persistent	Permanent
Recurrent AF episodes Terminate spontaneously within 7 days	AF that lasts longer than 7 days or requires termination (pharmacological/ electrical cardioversion)	AF that is refractory to cardioversion AF is the final rhythm as sinus rhythm cannot be restored.

EPIDEMIOLOGY
AF is increasingly common and has a prevalence of 1%–2% in the UK. Risk factors for developing AF include previous AF, increasing age, acute illness or any of the causes of AF (see the following section).

AETIOLOGY
A number of conditions cause AF:

Cardiac
- Hypertension
- IHD
- Valvular disease (e.g. mitral stenosis)
- Cardiomyopathy

Respiratory
- Pneumonia
- PE
- Pleural effusion
- Lung Ca

Endocrine
- Thyrotoxicosis
- Diabetes mellitus

Other
- Infection
- Drugs (thyroxine)
- Alcohol
- Electrolyte disturbance

PATHOLOGY
- Disruption of the electrical activity of the atria leads to rapid and chaotic contractions of the atria.
- As pulse rate increases the time for diastolic filling decreases, which may lead to a reduced cardiac output.

CLINICAL PRESENTATION
AF may be asymptomatic with the only clinical finding being an irregularly irregular pulse. Symptoms of AF include palpitations, shortness of breath, angina and presyncope.

EXAMINATION
Cardiovascular examination reveals an irregularly irregular pulse. If cardiovascular compromise → hypotension.

May be signs of concurrent/precipitant disease (thyrotoxicosis, pneumonia, valvular heart disease).

INVESTIGATIONS
- Bedside: BP, ECG (reveals absent p waves and an irregularly irregular rate).
- Bloods: FBC (↑WCC), CRP (infection), U&Es (electrolyte imbalance), TFTs (↑T3), lipids, bone profile (↑Ca^{2+}), glucose. If ACS suspected, check troponin. If PE suspected, check d-dimer.
- Imaging: CXR (respiratory pathology), echocardiogram (valvular disease).

DIFFERENTIAL DIAGNOSIS
The other cause of an irregularly irregular pulse is multiple ventricular ectopics. You can distinguish between multiple ectopics and AF by getting the patient to exercise; exercising causes ectopics to disappear.

MANAGEMENT
If the patient shows signs of **haemodynamic compromise**, seek senior help immediately.

Manage using an ABCDE approach and manage shock (oxygen, IV access). Attempt DC cardioversion; if unsuccessful then use IV amiodarone ± further cardioversion.

If the patient is haemodynamically stable:

Non-pharmacological
- If patient has obvious underlying precipitant (e.g. pneumonia) manage this initially
- Educate the patient about the condition and inform them that they must inform the DVLA if AF affects their ability to drive

Pharmacological (see *Table 1.6.1*)
- Rate control:
  - **Beta-blocker** or a **rate-limiting calcium channel blocker** (CCB) (diltiazem)
  - Choice between either a beta-blocker or CCB depends on comorbidities (beta-blockers contraindicated in existing heart failure or asthma)
  - **Digoxin** can be considered if beta-blockers or CCBs do not manage AF, or can be considered first-line in sedentary elderly patients with persistent or permanent AF

- If patient presents <48 hours, consider referral to hospital for consideration of cardioversion
- Rhythm control:
  - Cardiologists can initiate electrical cardioversion or pharmacological cardioversion if necessary
  - Drugs used for pharmacological cardioversion include **amiodarone** and **sotalol**
- Anticoagulation:
  - Assess stroke risk using **CHA$_2$DS$_2$VASc score** (see the following section):
    - If patient willing to take anticoagulant and score enough on the CHA$_2$DS$_2$VASc score → prescribe either **warfarin** or a novel oral anticoagulant drug (**NOAC**) such as dabigatran, rivaroxaban or apixaban
    - If warfarin is prescribed, an INR of 2–3 is the recommended target range
  - Assess bleeding risk using the **HAS-BLED score**
  - If anticoagulation is contraindicated, a combination of aspirin and clopidogrel can be offered

CHA$_2$DS$_2$VASc score (offer anticoagulation to all patients scoring 2 or men with a score of 1)
- **C**ongestive heart failure = 1
- **H**ypertension = 1
- **A**ge ≥75 years = 2
- **D**iabetes mellitus = 1
- **S**troke/TIA/thromboembolism = 2
- **V**ascular disease = 1
- **A**ge 65–74 years = 1
- **S**ex **c**ategory (female) = 1

COMPLICATIONS OF AF
- Thromboembolic events (such as ischaemic stroke)
- Heart failure
- Reduced quality of life
- Drug side effects

Table 1.6.1 Medications used in the management of AF

Medication	Mechanism of action	Side effects	Notes
Warfarin	Inhibits vitamin K-dependent synthesis of clotting factors	Bleeding Teratogen (avoid in prengnacy)	Requires frequent blood tests High INR can be reversed by vitamin K
Dabigatran	Direct thrombin inhibitor	Bleeding	High INR cannot be reversed
Rivaroxaban/apixiban	Factor Xa inhibitors	Bleeding	High INR cannot be reversed
Beta-blockers	Block beta-adrenergic receptors to reduce heart rate	Bradycardia, hypotension, nightmares	Non-cardioselective Can mask hypoglycaemia → choose cardioselective in diabetics
Diltiazem (CCB)	Blocks calcium channels to decrease heart rate and contractility	Hypotension, headache, constipation, swollen ankles	Avoid combination of beta-blocker and diltiazem (severe bradycardia)
Digoxin	Blocks myocardial Na$^+$/K$^+$ ATPase	Toxicity, gynaecomastia	Toxicity classically caused by ↓ K$^+$
Amiodarone	Class III antiarrhythmic	Photosensitivity, pneumonitis, thyroid disturbance	ECG, TFTs, LFTs, U&Es and CXR needed before treatment started

CARDIOLOGY: QUESTIONS

1.1 ACUTE CORONARY SYNDROME

1. What are the risk factors for an acute coronary syndrome?

2. Outline the initial prehospital management for an acute coronary syndrome.

3. What are the complications of a myocardial infarction?

1.2 HEART FAILURE

1. Name three signs of both left-sided and right-sided heart failure that you may elicit on examination.

2. How do you manage a patient presenting with acute pulmonary oedema?

3. Which drugs have been shown to reduce mortality in patients with chronic heart failure?

1.3 HYPERTENSION

1. What conservative and medical treatments would you consider for the management of a 56-year-old Caucasian woman with stage 2 hypertension?

2. Which investigations would you perform to look for evidence of end-organ damage in a hypertensive patient?

1.4 VALVULAR HEART DISEASE

1. What features may you find on cardiovascular examination in a patient with aortic stenosis?

2. What features may you find on cardiovascular examination in a patient with mitral regurgitation?

3. How would a patient with symptomatic aortic stenosis present in comparison to a patient with symptomatic mitral regurgitation?

1.5 INFECTIVE ENDOCARDITIS

1. Which organisms most commonly cause infective endocarditis?

2. What signs may you elicit on examination in patients with infective endocarditis?

3. Outline the two major Duke criteria for diagnosis of infective endocarditis.

1.6 ATRIAL FIBRILLATION

1. Name three causes of atrial fibrillation.

2. What ECG features are suggestive of atrial fibrillation?

3. What are the initial options available to rate control a patient with atrial fibrillation, providing no contraindications?

CHAPTER 2

Respiratory

2.1 ASTHMA

DEFINITION

Asthma is a chronic inflammatory condition of the respiratory system secondary to hypersensitivity, characterised by reversible airway obstruction, bronchospasm and smooth muscle hyperplasia.

EPIDEMIOLOGY

Asthma is a common condition with estimates suggesting 5.4 million people in the UK are receiving treatment.

AETIOLOGY

The fundamental causes of asthma are not known but a combination of genetic and environmental factors is thought to contribute. Irritants in the environment are thought to irritate the airway and provoke allergic reactions when susceptible patients are exposed to them.

Risk factors include:

● History (personal or family) of atopy (may be related to other IgE-mediated conditions, e.g. eczema)

● Allergen exposure: Indoor allergens (e.g. dust mites) or outdoor allergens (pollens/tobacco smoke)

● Occupation: Chemical irritants in the workplace (e.g. flour dust/isocyanates from paint)

● Outdoor cold air/exercise/extreme emotional arousal can trigger asthma

● Medications: NSAIDs, aspirin, beta-blockers have the potential to trigger asthma in susceptible patients

● A small subset of patients is affected by aspirin sensitivity – these patients exhibit Samter's triad (asthma/aspirin sensitivity/nasal polyps)

PATHOLOGY

The airways of asthma patients are hypersensitive and respond to triggers (usually via a type 1 hypersensitivity reaction). This hypersensitivity reaction leads to spasm of the bronchioles, causing constriction of the smooth muscle and inflammation of the airway. The increased work of the smooth muscle leads to hyperplasia within the bronchioles.

CLINICAL PRESENTATION

Patients with asthma can present acutely with features of acute asthma or more indolently with features of shortness of breath, cough (typically nocturnal) or audible wheeze.

EXAMINATION

Your examination will help you determine the severity of the asthma exacerbation (Figure 2.1.1).

Signs on examination may include:

● Increased respiratory effort ($\uparrow$ RR)

● Tachypnoea

● Widespread expiratory wheeze

INVESTIGATIONS

Bedside: Peak expiratory flow (PEF) (in the form of a bronchodilator reversibility test), spirometry (obstructive picture), fractional exhaled nitric oxide (FeNO) testing (if normal spirometry or negative bronchodilator reversibility test).

Bloods: FBC (eosinophilia/infection), CRP (infection), BNP (to help exclude heart failure if suspected). Consider ABG in acute asthma to check PaO_2 and $PaCO_2$.

Imaging: CXR (rule out other respiratory pathology causing shortness of breath).

DIFFERENTIAL DIAGNOSIS

The differential diagnosis for asthma includes COPD (see Section 2.2), bronchiectasis, GORD, heart failure (see Section 1.2), interstitial lung disease (see Section 2.4), lung cancer (see Section 2.5), pulmonary embolism, upper airway cough syndrome or infection such as pneumonia/TB.

Moderate Acute Asthma	Life-Threatening Asthma
Increasing symptoms	Any of:
PEF >50%–75% best or predicted	- PEF <33% best or predicted
No features of acute severe asthma	- SpO_2 <92%
	- PaO_2 <8kPa
	- Normal $PaCO_2$ (4.6–6.0 kPa)
	- Silent chest
Acute Severe Asthma	- Cyanosis
Any of:	- Poor respiratory effort
- PEF 33%–50% of best or predicted	- Arrhythmia
- RR >25/min	- Exhaustion
- Heart rate >110/min	- Altered conscious level
Inability to complete sentences in one breath	- Hypotension

Figure 2.1.1 Grading the severity of acute asthma.

MANAGEMENT
New diagnosis of asthma

The diagnostic testing for asthma in adults includes having spirometry with a bronchodilator reversibility test and an FeNO test.

- FeNO levels are raised when there is increased inflammation (as one type of NO rises in inflammatory cells, particularly eosinophils) and therefore the levels of FeNO correlate with the level of inflammation in the airway. A level of >40 parts per billion is considered positive
- Spirometry should show a FEV1/FVC ratio of <70% (an obstructive picture), which corresponds with obstructive lung diseases, such as asthma
- Reversibility testing in adults is positive if an improvement in FEV1 of 12% or more and an increase in volume of 200 mL or more is demonstrated in peak flow following use of a short-acting beta-2-agonist (SABA)

Acute asthma management

Patients should be managed via an ABCDE approach and categorised based on the severity of their asthma.

Observations, PEF, pulse oximetry and blood gases are needed to categorise a patient's asthma severity.

Patients with any features of life-threatening or severe asthma that are persistent despite treatment should be admitted to hospital. The treatment of acute asthma can be remembered by the mnemonic **SONS**: **S**teroids, **O**xygen, **N**ebulisers (salbutamol/ipratropium bromide), Magnesium **S**ulphate (can be used if patients have not had a good initial response to salbutamol therapy).

Intravenous aminophylline is also used in clinical practice but there is little evidence to support its use.

If a patient demonstrates features of worsening PEF/hypoxia or hypercapnia/exhaustion, then they should be considered for intensive care referral.

Chronic disease management
Non-pharmacological

- Educate about the condition and provide information on inhaler technique
- Address and identify triggers to the patient's asthma
- Lifestyle modifications (weight loss, smoking cessation) if appropriate
- Assess baseline status using a validated Control Questionnaire and provide a Personalised Asthma Action Plan
- Provide a peak flow meter

Pharmacological

Table 2.1.1 provides examples of medical management.

- Provide a SABA to all patients with symptomatic asthma

Table 2.1.1 Examples of medications used in asthma

Medication	Example	Side effects
Short-acting beta-2-agonist (SABA)	Salbutamol	Tachycardia, hypokalaemia, tremor
Short-acting muscarinic antagonist (SAMA)	Ipratropium	Dry mouth, cough, urinary retention, constipation
Long-acting beta-2-agonist (LABA)	Formoterol	As for SABA
Long-acting muscarinic antagonist (LAMA)	Tiotropium	Dry mouth, cough, urinary retention, constipation
Corticosteroids (ICS)	Beclometasone	Oral thrush, dry mouth, Cushing syndrome
Combination (ICS + LABA)	Fostair®/ Seretide®	As for ICS and LABA
Leukotriene receptor antagonist (LTRA)	Montelukast	Headache, eosinophilia, ↑ risk of eosinophilic granulomatosis with polyangiitis

- Further treatment for asthma can be given via a stepwise approach:
  - Step 1: SABA + low-dose inhaled corticosteroid (ICS)
  - Step 2: SABA + low-dose ICS + leukotriene receptor antagonist (LTRA)
  - Step 3: SABA + low-dose ICS + long-acting beta-2-agonist (LABA) + continue LTRA if responsive
  - Step 4: Change the ICS/LABA to a maintenance and reliever therapy (MART), which consists of a combination inhaler of ICS and fast-acting LABA
  - Step 5: Increase ICS to a moderate maintenance dose
  - Step 6: Increase ICS to high-dose OR trial of additional drug (e.g. theophylline, long-acting muscarinic receptor antagonist) OR refer to a specialist
- Omalizumab (autoantibody to IgE) is recommended for treating severe persistent confirmed allergic IgE-mediated asthma as an add-on therapy if a patient requires more than four courses of corticosteroids per year

REFERENCE

National Institute for Health and Care Excellence. Stepwise treatment. Adapted from NICE Guidelines on Asthma. https://www.nice.org.uk/guidance/ng80

2.2 CHRONIC OBSTRUCTIVE PULMONARY DISEASE

DEFINITION

Chronic obstructive pulmonary disease (COPD) is a chronic progressive respiratory disorder characterised by airway obstruction with little to no reversibility. It is an umbrella term that describes the damage to the airway caused by chronic bronchitis and emphysema.

EPIDEMIOLOGY

Current estimates suggest that more than three million people have COPD in the UK, with only one million of these being diagnosed.

AETIOLOGY

Smoking is by far the biggest aetiological factor for the development of COPD. Not all smokers develop COPD, suggesting that there are additional environmental or genetic factors that lead to the development of the condition. In a small number of people, COPD develops due to alpha-1 antitrypsin deficiency.

PATHOLOGY

COPD encompasses chronic bronchitis and emphysema.

Chronic bronchitis is a disease of the airway and is defined as inflammation of the bronchioles. It leads to goblet cell hyperplasia, chronic inflammation and fibrosis and mucus hypersecretion. Chronic bronchitis can be diagnosed with a **cough + sputum on most days for 3 months of 2 successive years**

Emphysema is a disease of the alveoli and is defined as the permanent dilation of airspaces distal to the terminal bronchiole. It is caused by the inflammatory process destroying elastin by activation of proteases. Without elastin, the alveoli are prone to collapse.

Patients with chronic bronchitis are classically referred to as 'Blue Bloaters' due to the increased sputum production that reduces alveolar ventilation.

Patients with emphysema are classically referred to a 'Pink Puffers'. This is because of their collapsed alveoli; they usually need to purse their lips to maintain a positive end expiratory pressure to keep the alveoli open in order to ventilate them.

The end result is that patients with COPD have ineffective removal of CO_2, leading to retention. Chronic CO_2 retention can lead to a respiratory acidosis, so the body compensates by producing more bicarbonate to neutralise this (look for it on the ABG!).

Types of COPD	
Blue Bloaters	Chronic bronchitis
Pink Puffers	Emphysema

CLINICAL PRESENTATION

Patients with COPD classically present with chronic productive cough and shortness of breath. Patients may also complain of an audible wheeze or side effects of CO_2 retention (such as drowsiness or confusion).

EXAMINATION

Patients with COPD may have a number of signs on examination:

Observations: ↑ RR, ↓ oxygen saturations.

Inspection: Pursed-lip breathing, use of accessory muscles of respiration; asterixis (CO_2 retention), hyperinflation (barrel chest), peripheral cyanosis.

Percussion: Hyper-resonant percussion note.

Auscultation: Widespread expiratory wheeze.

Features of cor pulmonale: Peripheral oedema, left parasternal heave, ↑ JVP, hepatomegaly.

INVESTIGATIONS

Bedside: Spirometry; include post-bronchodilator (confirms diagnosis), ECG (cor pulmonale), sputum culture.

Bloods: FBC (infection/secondary polycythaemia), BNP (exclude CCF), ABG (respiratory failure).

Imaging: CXR (exclude other respiratory pathology).

DIFFERENTIAL DIAGNOSIS

The differential diagnosis for COPD includes: Asthma (see Section 2.1), bronchiectasis, heart failure (see Section 1.2), lung cancer (see Section 2.5), interstitial lung disease (see Section 2.4), anaemia (see Section 8.1) or infection (e.g. pneumonia/TB).

MANAGEMENT

Acute exacerbations of COPD (AECOPD)

Exacerbations of COPD are most commonly caused by infections (most frequently *Haemophilus influenzae*, *Streptococcus pneumoniae* or *Moraxella catarrhalis*).

Patients should be managed with an ABCDE approach and oxygen saturations should be targeted at 88%–92%.

Medical management includes oxygen, nebulisers (short-acting beta-2-agonist and short-acting muscarinic antagonist) and corticosteroids. Antibiotics should be given for infective exacerbations (recommended if sputum is purulent or there are clinical signs of pneumonia).

For patients in decompensated type 2 respiratory failure that persists despite optimal medical therapy, non-invasive ventilation (NIV) is indicated. This helps correct the ventilation and oxygenation issues in AECOPD.

The DECAF score can be used as a prognostic score (0–6) for patients with AECOPD as a predictor of mortality:

- Dyspnoea (MRCD scale): Too breathless to leave the house (5a = 1) or wash or dress independently (5b = 2)
- Eosinopenia (<0.05) = 1
- Consolidation (present on CXR) = 1
- Acidaemia: ABG pH <7.35 = 1
- Fibrillation (evidence of atrial fibrillation) = 1

Asthma/steroid responsive features
- Atopy
- Eosinophilia
- Diurnal variation in PEF

Chronic disease management
Non-pharmacological
- Education about the condition
- Smoking cessation and pulmonary rehabilitation
- Multidisciplinary team approach (e.g. respiratory nurse, chest physiotherapy)
- Vaccinations (annual influenza, one-off pneumococcal)

Pharmacological
- Medical treatment of COPD follows a stepwise treatment ladder:
  - Step 1: Short-acting beta-2-agonist (SABA) or short-acting muscarinic antagonist (SAMA) PRN
  - Step 2:
    - If features of asthma or steroid responsiveness (see box)
      - ‡ Consider LABA + ICS (e.g. Duoresp®)
      - ‡ If still breathless, consider triple therapy with LAMA + LABA + ICS in a combination inhaler (e.g. Trelegy®)
    - If no features of asthma or steroid responsiveness:
      - ‡ Offer LABA + LAMA (e.g. Ultibro®)
- Other medical treatments include oral theophylline, mucolytics and long-term oxygen therapy (LTOT)
- For patients with frequent infective exacerbations of COPD (>4 per year requiring hospitalisation), azithromycin can be offered as prophylaxis providing the patient does not smoke. A sputum culture and CT scan is required prior to starting to rule out atypical organisms or *Pseudomonas* spp. and other lung pathology, respectively
- Roflumilast (phosphodiesterase-4 enzyme inhibitor) can be used as an add-on therapy for patients if they have an FEV1 <50% and had two or more AECOPD in 12 months despite triple therapy
- Offer LTOT to patients with a pO_2 of <7.3 kPa or to those with a pO_2 of 7.3–8 kPa and either secondary polycythaemia, nocturnal hypoxaemia, peripheral oedema or pulmonary hypertension
- If patients have chronic hypercapnic respiratory failure and have needed NIV, they can be referred for consideration of long-term NIV

Surgical
- Lung volume reduction surgery can be considered if the patient does not smoke, has an FEV1 <50% despite optimal medical treatment and can walk 140 metres in 6 minutes.

REFERENCE
National Institute for Health and Care Excellence. NICE guidelines on COPD. https://www.nice.org.uk/guidance/ng115

2.3 PNEUMONIA

DEFINITION

Pneumonia describes any inflammatory condition affecting the alveoli of the lung. In the vast majority of cases this is secondary to a bacterial infection. It can be classified by whether the illness started in the community (community-acquired pneumonia [CAP]) or after 48 hours in the hospital (hospital-acquired pneumonia [HAP]).

Technically, pneumonia is a radiological diagnosis following the identification of consolidation of a CXR.

EPIDEMIOLOGY

Pneumonia is a common condition affecting 5–10 people per 1000 adults in the UK each year. It is the condition responsible for more hospital admissions and bed days than any other respiratory condition in the UK.

AETIOLOGY

The vast majority of pneumonias are caused by a bacterial infection (*Table 2.3.1*). Occasionally, pneumonia may occur secondary to viral or fungal infection. The two most common organisms causing CAP are *Streptococcus pneumoniae* and *Haemophilus influenzae*. Bacterial organisms causing CAP can be further subdivided into **typical** and **atypical** organisms. Atypical organisms include *Mycoplasma pneumoniae* and *Legionella pneumophila*, which manifest in a number of systemic features.

Risk factors for the development of pneumonia include smoking, alcohol abuse, being underweight and comorbid conditions that may impact on normal lung function or clearance mechanisms, such as chronic respiratory diseases, cardiovascular disease, cerebrovascular disease, dementia, Parkinson disease, dysphagia, CKD, HIV and chronic liver disease.

PATHOLOGY

Depending on the causative organism, pneumonias are generally transmitted from inhalation airborne microbes. The organisms invade the spaces between cells and alveoli and cause an inflammatory response to occur, with the formation of pus, bacteria and inflammatory cells usually confined within a lobe of the lung.

CLINICAL PRESENTATION

Patients with pneumonia present with shortness of breath, productive cough and potentially fever and pleuritic chest pain. There may be extra features of the underlying organisms (e.g. rash secondary to streptococcal infection). Patients may present acutely unwell with sepsis secondary to their pneumonia and may be in shock.

EXAMINATION

Examination findings for patients with pneumonia include signs of increased respiratory effort (↑ RR), tachycardia and fever. Auscultation findings include reduced breath sounds, bronchial breathing, increased tactile fremitus and vocal resonance and crackles over the affected area.

INVESTIGATIONS

Bedside; Sputum culture (if productive), ECG (tachycardia or if pleuritic chest pain), urine sample (for uri-

Table 2.3.1 Organisms that can cause pneumonia

Organism	Class	Clinical circumstances
Streptococcus pneumoniae	Gram positive diplococci	Most common pneumonia (70%) Classically causes reactivation of herpes simplex virus in 1/3 of cases
Haemophilus influenzae	Gram negative coccobaccilus	More common in patients with preexisting lung disease and COPD
Moraxella catarrhalis	Gram negative diplococci	Occurs in COPD patients
Chlamydia psittaci, C. pneumoniae	Gram negative cocci	Occurs after prolonged contact with birds carrying *C. psittaci* (e.g. parrots)
Legionella pneumophila	Gram negative coccobaccilus	Classically occurs after being exposed to a faulty air conditioner/foreign pool Features include: Hyponatraemia (secondary to SIADH), pancreatitis, glomerulonephritis
Mycoplasma pneumoniae	Gram negative spindle	Classically occurs with systemic manifestations of erythema multiforme/ nodosum, haemolytic anaemia, arthritis Associated with Guillain-Barré syndrome
Staphlococcus aureus	Gram positive cocci	Classically occurs after influenza infection
Pneumocystis jirovecii	Yeast-like fungus	Immunocompromised patients (HIV/AIDS)

nary antigens such as *Pneumococcus* and *Legionella* spp.).

Bloods: FBC (infection), U&Es (check for dehydration and urea is used for prognostic information), CRP (inflammation), ABG (check for respiratory failure); blood cultures and lactate if septic.

Imaging: CXR (a CXR with consolidation is necessary for the diagnosis of pneumonia as it is a radiological diagnosis).

DIFFERENTIAL DIAGNOSIS

The differential diagnosis for pneumonia includes asthma (see Section 2.1), acute exacerbation of COPD (see Section 2.2), heart failure (see Section 1.2), lung cancer (see Section 2.5), pulmonary embolism, post-infectious cough, GORD or tuberculosis.

MANAGEMENT

The management of patients with CAP is determined by a risk stratification process called the CURB-65 (*Table 2.3.2*).

(Note that in primary care a version of the CURB-65 is used, the **CRB-65**, as access to an immediate urea result will not be available in order to help clinical decision making.)

- Patients with a CURB-65 score of 0 should be managed in the community with amoxicillin (unless penicillin allergic)

Table 2.3.2 CURB-65 score

C	Confusion (abbreviated mental state score ≤8)
U	Urea >7 mmol/L
R	Respiratory rate ≥30/min
B	Blood pressure ≤90 mmgHg systolic or ≤60 mmHg diastolic
65	Age ≥65 years

- Patients with a CURB-65 score of 1 can be managed in the community with a combination of antibiotic therapy (amoxicillin + clarithromycin) or monotherapy with doxycycline if their oxygen saturations are >92%
- Patients with a CURB-65 score of 2 are usually managed in hospital with oral combination antibiotic therapy or doxycycline monotherapy (as stated previously)
- Patients with a CURB-65 of >2 are managed in hospital usually with IV antibiotics as this represents a severe CAP

Other non-pharmacological management strategies may help alleviate symptoms, such as hot water, lemon soothers and stopping smoking.

2.4 INTERSTITIAL LUNG DISEASE

DEFINITION

Interstitial lung disease (ILD) is a term used to describe a number of conditions characterised by inflammation and progressive fibrosis of the airways.

EPIDEMIOLOGY

The most common ILD is idiopathic pulmonary fibrosis (IPF), which has an estimated incidence of 7 per 100,000 people in the UK.

AETIOLOGY/PATHOLOGY

There are a number of different causes for ILD. The source of the fibrosis can help identify the underlying cause.

Causes

- Infection: TB, atypical pneumonia
- Inhaled: Silicosis, asbestosis, berylliosis (inorganic), extrinsic allergic alveolitis (organic)
- Idiopathic: IPF, sarcoidosis, antisynthetase syndrome
- Malignancy: Lymphangitis carcinomatosa
- Connective tissue disease: SLE, RA, dermatomyositis, polymyositis, systemic sclerosis
- Drugs: Nitrofurantoin, methotrexate, amiodarone, sulfasalazine, simvastatin

---

Extrinsic allergic alveolitis

Also known as hypersensitivity pneumonitis.

Caused by inflammatory reaction to inhaled organic particles due to a type III hypersensitivity reaction.

Examples:

Bird-fancier's lung: *Chlamydia psittaci*

Malt-worker's lung: *Aspergillus clavatus*

Farmer's lung: Spores from *Saccharopolyspora rectivirgula*

Sugar worker's lung: *Thermoactinomyces sacchari*

Despite the variety of causes of ILD, they all have the potential to cause prolonged inflammation in the lungs and progressive fibrosis. As a result of this fibrosis, the lungs become scarred and thickened, making it more difficult for proficient oxygenation to occur (*Table 2.4.1*).

IPF is labelled as the cause of ILD when no other cause can be identified.

CLINICAL PRESENTATION

ILD classically presents with a dry cough and shortness of breath that is worsened on exertion. Patients may also have symptoms and signs suggestive of the underlying cause.

Table 2.4.1 Causes of obstructive and restrictive spirometry results

Obstructive	Restrictive
$\downarrow\downarrow$ FEV1	$\downarrow$ FEV1
$\downarrow$ FVC	$\downarrow\downarrow$ FVC
$\downarrow$ FEV1:FVC ratio ($<$0.7)	$\uparrow$ FEV1:FVC ratio ($>$0.8)
Causes: Asthma, COPD, bronchiectasis, cystic fibrosis	Causes: Interstitial lung disease, sarcoidosis, obesity

EXAMINATION

Examination findings may include increased respiratory effort, clubbing and fine end-inspiratory crackles.

Crackles occur both in pneumonia and in ILD. To distinguish between the two, ask the patient to cough. If the crackles change or disappear following a cough, then the cause is more likely to be due to pneumonia rather than ILD, where the crackles do not change following a cough. This is due to the underlying mechanism causing the crackles. In an infectious cause, the crackles are caused by pus from the causative organism that can move around the airway, whereas fibrotic lungs cannot move around as freely.

Cor pulmonale

Cor pulmonale refers to enlargement and failure of the right side of the heart as a result of increased vascular resistance in the lungs, usually secondary to pathology such as ILD or COPD.

Right ventricular hypertrophy can occur.

ECG finds include:

- Right axis deviation (positive lead I and negative aVF)
- p Pulmonale (peaked p waves indicate right atrial enlargement)
- Right ventricular hypertrophy (dominant R wave in V1 and dominant S wave in V5/6)

Treatment options include LTOT, diuretics for right heart failure and vasodilators (e.g. nifedipine). Transplant can be used in extreme circumstances.

INVESTIGATIONS

Bedside: ECG (cor pulmonale), spirometry (restrictive picture).

Bloods: FBC (anaemia/infection), bone profile ($\uparrow$ Ca^{2+} in sarcoidosis), immunological profile (screen for underlying autoimmune case), ABG (respiratory failure).

Imaging: CXR (shows fibrosis, exclude other causes), high-resolution CT scan (honeycombing of the lung), transfer factor (↓ TLCO).

In addition to the previously presented findings, IPF has a positive ANA in 30% and rheumatoid factor in 10% of cases, although this does not necessarily mean that the ILD is secondary to a connective tissue disease.

DIFFERENTIAL DIAGNOSIS

The differential diagnosis for ILD includes asthma (see Section 2.1), COPD (see Section 2.2), heart failure (see Section 1.2), lung cancer (see Section 2.5), anaemia (see Section 8.1) and bronchiectasis.

MANAGEMENT

Chronic disease
Non-pharmacological
- Educate about the condition
- Address lifestyle factors and stop smoking if relevant
- Address risk factors for development of complications (e.g. right heart failure)
- Multidisciplinary approach including pulmonary rehabilitation

Pharmacological
Few medications have shown benefit in ILD.
- For IPF, the antifibrotic agent pirfenidone is recommended by NICE for patients who have an FVC of between 50% and 80% of predicted
- The tyrosine-kinase inhibitor nintedanib is also recommended by NICE to treat patients with IPF who have an FVC of between 50% and 80% of predicted
- For many patients, long-term oxygen therapy is necessary

Surgical
- Lung transplantation may be required for patients with severe fibrosis

SITE OF FIBROSIS

Some conditions predominantly cause fibrosis either in the upper or lower zones of the lung. This can be useful to know when looking at x-rays or answering examination questions.

Upper zone fibrosis
- Extrinsic allergic alveolitis
- Inhaled inorganic molecules (silicosis, berylliosis)
- TB
- Ankylosing spondylitis (see XXX)
- Sarcoidosis

Lower zone fibrosis
- Idiopathic pulmonary fibrosis
- Connective tissue disorders (except ankylosing spondylitis)
- Drug-induced fibrosis
- Asbestosis

Sarcoidosis: Multisystem granulomatous disorder of unknown cause. Most common in northern Europe in 20–40 year age bracket. Clinical features include polyarthralgia, erythema nodosum and bilateral hilar lymphadenopathy. Blood tests may show a raised calcium and serum ACE. Treatment is with corticosteroids and immunosuppression.

Systemic sclerosis: Connective tissue disease characterised by hardened, sclerotic skin. Can occur with skin tightening alone (scleroderma) or with systemic involvement (limited or diffuse). Limited cutaneous systemic sclerosis is associated with Raynaud phenomenon, predominant face and limb involvement and positive anti-centromere antibodies. CREST syndrome (calcinosis, Raynaud phenomenon, oesophageal dysmotility, sclerodactyly, telangiectasia) is a subtype of limited cutaneous systemic sclerosis. Diffuse cutaneous systemic sclerosis affects the trunk and proximal limbs predominantly, as well as the lungs and kidneys. Associated with positive scl-70 antibodies.

Polymyositis: Inflammatory muscle disorder that is either idiopathic or associated with other connective tissue diseases or malignancy. Features include proximal muscle weakness, Raynaud phenomenon and ILD. Investigations show a ↑ CK and positive anti-Jo1 antibodies. Dermatomyositis is a variant that involves the skin, manifesting in purple papules on the knuckles (Gottron) and a purple heliotrope rash around the eyes.

2.5 LUNG CANCER

DEFINITION

Lung cancers are malignant tumours in the lung parenchyma. Some types affect the airway (small cell, non-small cell) and others affect the pleura (mesothelioma).

EPIDEMIOLOGY

Lung cancer accounts for 20% of all cancers in the UK and is the leading cause of death among cancers in the UK. Non-small cell lung cancer (NSCLC) is the most common type of lung cancer.

AETIOLOGY

Smoking is the biggest aetiological factor for the development of lung cancer. Other risk factors include occupational exposures (asbestos, chromium and radiation).

PATHOLOGY

Exposure to carcinogens in the air (such as cigarette smoke) cause genetic mutations (e.g. in p53) leading to the creation of malignant cells. Lung cancers can develop from a number of cell types, leading to separate histological classifications.

- **Epithelial cell** origin leads to the formation of non-small cell lung cancer. There are three types of non-small cell lung cancer:
  - Squamous cell lung cancer: Central tumours associated with finger clubbing and hypercalcaemia from parathyroid hormone-related protein (PTHrP) secretion
  - Adenocarcinoma: Peripheral tumours that are the most common lung cancer in non-smokers
  - Large cell lung carcinoma: Peripheral tumours that are poorly differentiated; they are associated with β-hCG secretion
- Neuroendocrine cell origin leads to the formation of small cell lung cancer. Small cell lung cancers are usually central and are associated with a number of paraneoplastic syndromes depending on the hormone secreted:
  - ADH → Hyponatraemia from SIADH
  - ACTH → Cushing syndrome
  - Antibodies to voltage gated calcium channels (Lambert–Eaton syndrome)

Mesotheliomas have a slightly different pathology. Asbestos exposure leads to the formation of plaques in the pleura. These plaques can undergo malignant transformation into a mesothelioma.

CLINICAL PRESENTATION

Patients with lung cancer classically present with symptoms of a persistent cough, haemoptysis and shortness of breath. They may also have chest pain and recurrent chest infections. Systemic symptoms (fatigue, weight loss) may be present, in addition to the symptoms of a paraneoplastic syndrome or metastasis (e.g. hypercalcaemia).

NICE Guidelines state that patients should be referred down the 2-week wait pathway for lung cancer if:

- They have CXR findings suggestive of lung cancer
- Are aged over 40 with unexplained haemoptysis

Additionally, an urgent CXR should be performed to assess for lung cancer in people >40 years if they have two or more of the following symptoms, or one of the following if they have ever smoked:

- Cough
- Fatigue
- Shortness of breath
- Chest pain
- Weight loss
- Appetite loss

EXAMINATION

Inspection: Cachexia, clubbing, hypertrophic pulmonary osteoarthropathy, acanthosis nigricans.

Respiratory examination: Lymphadenopathy, lung collapse/consolidation, pleural effusion.

Additionally, patients may present with complications of lung cancer and have the following signs on examination:

- Horner syndrome (Pancoast tumour – an apical lung tumour compression of the sympathetic chain)
- Fatiguability and bilateral ptosis (Lambert–Eaton syndrome)
- Dermatomyositis (Gottron papules and periorbital oedema)
- Cushingoid (see Section 4.4)

INVESTIGATIONS

Bedside: ECG, sputum culture (if productive).

Bloods: FBC (anaemia), U&Es ($\downarrow$ Na$^+$), bone profile ($\uparrow$ Ca^{2+}), LFTs ($\uparrow$ ALP).

Imaging: CXR, CT scan (staging), radionucleotide bone scan (for metastases), PET scanning (for NSCLC).

Invasive: Pleural fluid analysis (exudate), bronchoscopy and tissue biopsy.

MANAGEMENT

All smokers should be encouraged to stop smoking.

Treatment for lung cancer is based on the type of tumour and its staging:

- NSCLC: Approximately 20% are suitable for surgical treatment in the form of lobectomy. Radiotherapy and chemotherapy are options in these patients.

Table 2.5.1 Comparing transudate vs. exudate pleural effusions

Transudate	Exudate
Caused by organ failure • Heart failure • Hepatic failure • Renal failure • Due to a low protein causing fluid to shift into the pleural space	Causes include Infection – Pneumonia/TB Malignancy – Lung cancer, mesothelioma Inflammation – Rheumatoid arthritis, CTD, vasculitis Other – Hypothyroidism, pancreatitis, Dressler syndrome
Protein typically <3 g/dL	Protein typically >3 g/dL

• SCLC: Usually metastatic at time of diagnosis. Patients with very early stage disease (T1–2a) can be considered for surgery. The majority of patients will receive a combination of chemotherapy and radiotherapy.

Causes of pleural effusions: Light's criteria can be used to distinguish between the two; it uses LDH and pH to differentiate between transudate and exudate pleural effusions (*Table 2.5.1*).

Pulmonary embolism (PE)

A PE is a blockage of the pulmonary arteries in the form of an embolus.

Having active cancer makes PEs more likely (due to disorganised angiogenesis from the cancer).

Patients may have features of DVT (red, warm, swollen, painful calf) prior to the features of a PE.

Clinical presentation

Clinical features include symptoms such as sudden onset shortness of breath, haemoptysis, pleuritic chest pain and palpitations.

Investigations

Bedside: ECG findings include sinus tachycardia (most commonly), right axis deviation, RBBB, S1Q3T3.

Bloods: D-dimer is non-specific but often raised in patients with a PE. Arterial blood gases show T1RF.

Imaging: CXRs are often clear (unless a provoking lung cancer is found). Imaging is used to confirm a PE using either a CTPA or a V/Q scan.

Management

Treatment involves giving either a high-dose LMWH or fondaparinux followed by 3–6 months of anticoagulation, usually in the form of warfarin/NOAC.

If a patient has evidence of haemodynamic instability (e.g. shock) with a PE, thrombolysis can be considered, usually with alteplase, in a high-dependency environment.

The length of anticoagulation depends on whether the PE was considered to be provoked (e.g. by cancer or long-distance travel) or unprovoked. If a PE was unprovoked, treatment is longer (usually 6 months). Investigations for cancer are recommended, e.g. FBC/LFTs/calcium/CXR and potentially a CT abdomen/pelvis.

REFERENCE

National Institute for Health and Care Excellence. NICE Guidelines for Lung Cancer: https://www.nice.org.uk/guidance/ng122

RESPIRATORY: QUESTIONS

2.1 ASTHMA

1. What are the risk factors for the development of asthma?
2. Which tests are performed for a new diagnosis of asthma?
3. Which medications are used in an acute exacerbation of asthma?

2.2 CHRONIC OBSTRUCTIVE PULMONARY DISEASE

1. What is the greatest aetiological factor for the development of COPD?
2. Which organisms commonly cause an infective exacerbation of COPD?
3. What are the management options for COPD?

2.3 PNEUMONIA

1. Which organisms commonly cause a community-acquired pneumonia?
2. What makes up the CURB-65 score for the management of community-acquired pneumonia?

2.4 INTERSTITIAL LUNG DISEASE

1. What are the causes of interstitial lung disease?
2. What is cor pulmonale and what are the ECG findings?
3. Which medications can be used to treat idiopathic pulmonary fibrosis?

2.5 LUNG CANCER

1. What are the presenting features of lung cancer?
2. What is the most common type of lung cancer?
3. What are the paraneoplastic syndromes that can occur with lung cancer?

Gastroenterology

3.1 CROHN'S DISEASE

DEFINITION

Crohn's disease is a form of inflammatory bowel disease. It is a chronic, relapsing, remitting, granulomatous condition that typically can affect any part of the gastrointestinal tract.

AETIOLOGY

The cause of Crohn's disease is unknown but suspected to be multifactorial. Risk factors include a family history of inflammatory bowel disease, previous infectious gastroenteritis, and drugs (NSAIDs). Smoking is a causative factor in Crohn's disease (two-thirds of sufferers are smokers, and smoking cessation halves the relapse rate) whereas smoking is protective in ulcerative colitis – this is one of many differentiating factors between the two diseases (see *Table 3.1.1*).

PATHOLOGY

There is transmural inflammation of the gastrointestinal tract (affecting all layers including the serosa). Crohn's disease most commonly affects the terminal ileum and colon (but can affect anywhere from mouth to anus). Inflammation leads to the development of granulomas. As the inflammation is transmural, patients with Crohn's may develop strictures, fistulas and adhesions.

CLINICAL PRESENTATION

Patients may present at any age but are more likely to develop symptoms in adolescence and early adulthood.

Diarrhoea and **abdominal pain** are prominent symptoms. Blood may be present in the stool if the patient has developed Crohn's colitis. Mucous may be present in the stool.

Other gastrointestinal symptoms include aphthous ulceration in the mouth and perianal skin tags.

Patients may also present with bowel obstruction (due to strictures) or perianal fistulas.

Non-specific symptoms include weight loss and lethargy. Malabsorption is common due to the involvement of the terminal ileum. Consider Crohn's disease in children who are 'failing to thrive'.

Extra-intestinal features of Crohn's disease are a commonly asked examination question. These can be remembered by the mnemonic **C-3P-O**, **C**lubbing, e**P**iscleritis, **P**yoderma gangrenosum/erythema nodosum, arthritis (**P**ainful joints), **O**steoporosis.

EXAMINATION

Abdominal examination may reveal tenderness or mass (commonly in the right lower quadrant due to the involvement of the terminal ileum).

Table 3.1.1 Features of inflammatory bowel disease (Crohn's disease vs. Ulcerative colitis)

	Crohn's disease	Ulcerative colitis
Risk factors	Smoking is a risk factor	Smoking is protective
Affected areas	Mouth → anus Terminal ileum most commonly affected Skip lesions Transmural inflammation	Ileocaecal valve → rectum Continuous lesions No inflammation beyond submucosa
GI symptoms	Diarrhoea ± blood/mucus RIF pain Mouth ulcers Bowel obstruction/fistulae Malabsorption	Diarrhoea + blood Lower abdominal pain Tenesmus Fecal urgency
Extra-intestinal symptoms	Arthritis/enteropathic arthritis Eye disease (most commonly episcleritis) Liver disease – Gallstones Other – Osteoporosis, amyloidosis, venous thromboembolism	Arthritis/enteropathic arthritis Eye disease (most commonly uveitis) Liver disease – PSC, autoimmune hepatitis Other – Venous thromboembolism
GI complications	Abscesses, intestinal strictures, bowel obstruction, fistula formation, perianal disease Colorectal cancer	Toxic megacolon (distended colon at risk of perforation) Colorectal cancer (↑ risk compared to Crohn's)

Rectal examination is required to identify any perianal lesions (skin tags, abscesses, fistulae).

A general examination should be performed looking for extra-intestinal manifestations.

INVESTIGATIONS

Bedside: Stool MC&S (exclude infection), fecal calprotectin (can help differentiate from IBS).

Bloods: FBC (anaemia, ↑ WCC), CRP/ESR (active inflammation), LFTs, vitamin B_{12}, D (deficiency).

Imaging: AXR (for evidence of bowel obstruction/proximal constipation/toxic megacolon in UC).

Invasive: Colonoscopy (to confirm diagnosis); features suggestive of Crohn's disease include deep ulcers and skip lesions.

DIFFERENTIAL DIAGNOSIS

The differential diagnosis for inflammatory bowel disease includes IBS, coeliac disease, gastroenteritis, diverticulitis, colonic tumour, pseudomembranous colitis and ischaemic colitis.

MANAGEMENT

Acute flare treatment

Emergency hospital admission should be arranged if the patient is systemically unwell with symptoms of bloody diarrhoea, fever, tachycardia or hypotension. This is managed with an ABCDE approach.

Exclude an alternative cause for diarrhoea symptoms (e.g. infection).

Glucocorticosteroids (e.g. IV hydrocortisone, oral prednisolone) are the mainstays of treatment for acute flares.

Budesonide can be considered if patients cannot tolerate a glucocorticosteroid or if they are contraindicated.

5-ASA treatments (e.g. mesalazine) can be used as add-on to glucocorticosteroids but are less effective.

If the flare of Crohn's is considered to be severe, then do not offer budesonide or 5-ASA drugs.

Biologics (infliximab, adalimumab) can be used in patients with a severe Crohn's flare as an add-on therapy.

Chronic disease management (maintaining remission)

Non-pharmacological

NICE Guidelines recommend the following be discussed with patients with Crohn's disease:

- Educate about the condition and about support groups available; screen for depression
- Provide smoking cessation advice
- Assess osteoporosis risk
- Offer colonoscopic surveillance (colorectal cancer)
- Monitor serum ferritin, vitamin B_{12}, folate, calcium and vitamin D levels
- Give information about the possible effects of Crohn's disease on pregnancy

Pharmacological

- 5-ASA agents are used to maintain remission as a first-line agent
- Methotrexate can be used as a second-line agent
- If on immunosuppressive or biologic therapy, ensure that patients receive influenza and pneumococcal vaccines
- Supplementation for ferritin, vitamin B_{12}, folate, calcium and vitamin D if necessary
- Supplementation to manage osteoporosis risk if necessary
- Diarrhoea can be treated symptomatically with codeine phosphate or loperamide unless due to active disease
- Avoid NSAIDs as can precipitate relapse

Surgical

80% of Crohn's patients will eventually require surgery. The most common procedure is an ileocaecal resection.

REFERENCE

National Institute for Health and Care Excellence. NICE Guidelines for Crohn's Disease. https://www.nice.org.uk/guidance/ng129

3.2 ULCERATIVE COLITIS

DEFINITION

Ulcerative colitis (UC) is a form of inflammatory bowel disease. It is a chronic, relapsing, remitting, condition that causes inflammation of the large bowel.

AETIOLOGY

The cause of UC is unknown but is suspected to be a combination of genetics (potentially HLA B27) and environment factors. There may be a family history of inflammatory bowel disease, colorectal cancer or coeliac disease. Smoking is a protective factor in UC (whereas it correlates with the risk of developing Crohn's disease).

PATHOLOGY

The inflammation in UC starts in the rectum (which is why this is the most common site for UC) and spreads proximally along the large bowel, but does not extend beyond the ileocaecal valve. Lesions are continuous. UC only affects the mucosa of the large bowel and hence causes superficial ulcers rather than granulomas (as seen in Crohn's). The widespread ulceration with preservation of adjacent mucosa can give the appearance of pseudopolyps. Inflammatory cells migrate through the walls of the GI tract to form crypt abscesses.

CLINICAL PRESENTATION

Bloody diarrhoea is the classic symptom of patients presenting with UC. Other features include urgency, tenesmus (urge to pass stool when the rectum is empty), abdominal pain (particularly in the lower left quadrant) and rectal bleeding. Patients may also present with non-specific symptoms such as weight loss, failure to thrive and fatigue. Extra-intestinal features include arthritis, uveitis, pyoderma gangrenosum or erythema nodosum and sclerosing cholangitis.

EXAMINATION

Abdominal examination: May reveal tenderness in the LIF.

Rectal examination: Required to identify any perianal lesions (skin tags, abscesses, fistulae).

A general examination should be performed looking for extra-intestinal manifestations.

INVESTIGATIONS

Bedside: Stool MC + S (exclude infection/*Clostridium difficile*), fecal calprotectin (can help differentiate from IBS).

Bloods: FBC (anaemia, ↑ WCC), CRP/ESR (active inflammation), LFTs, renal profile, tissue transglutaminase (exclude coeliac), TMPT (if needed; see box).

Imaging: AXR (for evidence of bowel obstruction/proximal constipation/toxic megacolon in UC).

Invasive: Colonoscopy (to confirm diagnosis).

> ### TMPT (thiopurine methyltransferase)
>
> Azathioprine is metabolised into its active form 6-MP. TMPT (thiopurine methyltransferase) is the enzyme that inactivates 6-MP.
>
> Patients with low or absent TMPT activity are at increased risk of bone marrow toxicity. Levels therefore need to be checked prior to starting azathioprine therapy.

DIFFERENTIAL DIAGNOSIS

The differential diagnosis for inflammatory bowel disease includes IBS, coeliac disease, gastroenteritis, diverticulitis, colonic tumour, pseudomembranous colitis and ischaemic colitis.

MANAGEMENT

Acute flare treatment

The severity of a UC flare needs to be assessed to guide management (*Table 3.2.1*).

In adults, emergency admission should be arranged if there are clinical features suggestive of severe ulcerative colitis.

Inducing remission

Mild/Moderate UC: Oral 5-ASA agent (e.g. mesalazine) + oral prednisolone. Consider topical 5-ASA if proctitis.

If no response to oral prednisolone in 2–4 weeks, consider adding oral tacrolimus.

Severe UC: IV hydrocortisone is the mainstay of treatment for acute severe flares.

Patients with acute UC flares are more likely to require surgery if any of the following are present:

- Stool frequency of more than eight per day
- Pyrexia

Table 3.2.1 Grading of severity in acute flares of ulcerative colitis

Severity	Symptoms
Mild	Less than four liquid stools/day Little/no rectal bleeding No signs of systemic disturbance
Moderate	Between four and six liquid stools/day Moderate rectal bleeding
Severe	More than six liquid stools/day Severe rectal bleeding Pyrexia >37.8, ↑ WCC Signs of shock (↑ pulse ↓ blood pressure) ↑ ESR (>30), ↓ Hb (<10.5)

- Tachycardia
- AXR showing colonic dilatation
- Low albumin, low haemoglobin, high platelet count or C-reactive protein (CRP) above 45 mg/L

Chronic disease management (maintaining remission)

Non-pharmacological

NICE Guidelines recommend the following be discussed with patients with ulcerative colitis:

- Educate about the condition and about support groups available; screen for depression
- Assess osteoporosis risk
- Offer colonoscopic surveillance (colorectal cancer)

Pharmacological

- 5-ASA agents are used to maintain remission
- Azathioprine or mercaptopurine can be used to maintain remission in patients who have had two or more exacerbations in <12 months or if remission is not maintained by aminosalicylates

- Supplementation to manage osteoporosis risk if necessary
- Avoid anti-diarrhoeal drugs as they can diminish colonic motility and may precipitate toxic megacolon

Surgical

- If patients are failing to respond to medical therapy, they should be considered for surgery
- If a patient has toxic megacolon, they require surgery
- Surgical options include a panproctocolectomy with subsequent ileostomy, or an initial total colectomy with ileostomy and rectal stump followed by being offered either an ileal reservoir or completion proctectomy

REFERENCE

National Institute for Health and Care Excellence. NICE Guidelines for Ulcerative Colitis. https://cks.nice.org.uk/ulcerative-colitis

3.3 COELIAC DISEASE

DEFINITION

Coeliac disease is an autoimmune disorder where chronic inflammation, malabsorption and damage to the lining of the small intestine occur in response to gluten-derived peptides.

EPIDEMIOLOGY

Coeliac disease affects approximately 1 in 100 people in the UK. It can affect people at any age but more commonly presents between 0–5 and 30–40 years of age. It is more common in women. Risk factors include a family history of coeliac disease (10%–15% of first-degree relatives) and a history of atopy and other autoimmune conditions, such as type 1 diabetes mellitus and Graves disease.

AETIOLOGY

The exact cause for the heightened immunological response to gluten as seen in coeliac disease is unknown. There is a strong immunological component to the condition as it occurs more commonly among people with other autoimmune diseases (such as type 1 diabetes mellitus). People can have a genetic predisposition to developing coeliac disease as there is a close association between the disease and human leukocyte antigens (HLAs), particularly HLA DQ2.

PATHOLOGY

Repeated exposure to gluten leads to villous atrophy of the small intestine and causes malabsorption. Villous atrophy along with crypt hyperplasia results in a smooth mucosal surface when viewed on histology.

CLINICAL PRESENTATION

Typical symptoms for coeliac disease include persistent gastrointestinal symptoms such as bloating, foul-smelling diarrhoea (due to malabsorption), indigestion and constipation.

Other presentations include:
- Weight loss
- Fatigue
- Unexplained iron/B_{12}/folate deficiency
- Failure to thrive in children

EXAMINATION

Clinical examination may be normal but may reveal:
- Aphthous ulceration
- Angular stomatitis (due to iron deficiency anaemia)
- Dermatitis herpetiformis (autoimmune blistering skin disorder caused by deposition of IgA associated with coeliac disease)
- Paraesthesia and polyneuropathy (folate/B_{12} deficiency)

> ### Subacute combined degeneration of the cord (SCDC)
>
> A neurological condition caused by B_{12} deficiency that results in degeneration of the dorsal columns and lateral corticospinal tracts, causing mixed UMN and LMN signs with ataxia.
>
> Where patients have both B_{12} and folate deficiency (as in coeliac disease), the B_{12} deficiency should be treated first so as to not precipitate SCDC.

INVESTIGATIONS

Coeliac disease should be tested for if a person has:
- Persistent, unexplained abdominal or gastrointestinal symptoms
- Faltering growth in children
- Prolonged fatigue
- Unexpected weight loss
- Severe or persistent mouth ulcers
- Unexplained iron, vitamin B_{12}, or folate deficiency
- Type 1 diabetes mellitus
- Autoimmune thyroid disease
- Irritable bowel syndrome in adults
- A first-degree relative with coeliac disease

Bedside: Stool MC + S (exclude infection/*C. difficile*), measure BMI to assess potential malnutrition.

Bloods: Tissue transglutaminase, total IgA, FBC (anaemia, ↑ WCC), CRP/ESR (active inflammation), TFTs (autoimmune thyroiditis), blood glucose (T1DM), LFTs (autoimmune hepatitis), vitamin B_{12}, D, folate and calcium screen for deficiency.

Invasive: Endoscopy and biopsy of the small intestine.

> ### Blood tests for coeliac disease
>
> Immunoglobulin A (IgA) tissue transglutaminase antibody (tTGA) and total IgA are first-line investigations.
>
> IgA endomysial antibody (EMA) can be used if IgA tTGA is unavailable, or in cases where it is weakly positive.
>
> If patients are already taking a gluten-free diet they should be asked, if possible, to reintroduce gluten for at least 6 weeks prior to testing.
>
> (NICE Guidelines 2016.)

DIFFERENTIAL DIAGNOSIS

Coeliac disease causes a range of symptoms and signs that can be caused by a variety of conditions, such as:

- Inflammatory bowel disease (see Sections 3.1, 3.2)
- Malignancy (gastrointestinal, haematological, ovarian)
- Infection (gastroenteritis, HIV/TB infection)
- Irritable bowel syndrome
- Cow's milk protein allergy (children)

MANAGEMENT

Chronic disease

Non-pharmacological

- Educate about the condition and advise about a gluten-free diet omitting:
  - Wheat (bread/pasta), barley (beer), rye and oats
- Assess osteoporosis risk
- Annual blood testing, including:
  - FBC and ferritin: Assess for anaemia
  - TFTs: Screen for autoimmune thyroiditis
  - LFTs: Screen for autoimmune hepatitis

- Vitamin D, B_{12}, folate and serum calcium: To assess for deficiency
- Renal profile: To assess for Addison's disease
- If the patient is pregnant or planning a pregnancy, offer folic acid 5 mg once daily
- Offer patients pneumococcal and influenza vaccine due to potential hyposplenism

COMPLICATIONS OF COELIAC DISEASE

- Anaemia (iron, folate, B_{12}): Folate deficiency is more common than B_{12} in coeliac disease
- Osteoporosis
- Hyposplenism
- Bacterial overgrowth
- Cancer such as Hodgkin and non-Hodgkin lymphoma
- Subfertility
- Lactose intolerance

REFERENCE

National Institute for Health and Care Excellence. NICE Guideline for Coeliac Disease. https://www.nice.org.uk/guidance/ng20

3.4 LIVER FAILURE

DEFINITION

Liver failure describes the spectrum of disease when the liver loses its ability to regenerate or repair.

It can occur acutely (acute liver failure) or following progress to cirrhosis. A number of terms are used to define the timing of liver failure: fulminant hepatic failure (FHF) describes failure that occurs within 8 weeks of onset of the underlying illness. Subacute FHF occurs within 8–26 weeks and chronic decompensated hepatic failure occurs over a period $\geq$6 months. Cirrhosis occurs when the liver is replaced by fibrotic tissue and represents the final histological pathway for a number of liver diseases.

EPIDEMIOLOGY

There are an estimated 30,000 patients in the UK with liver cirrhosis, with nearly one-third diagnosed as new cases annually.

AETIOLOGY/PATHOLOGY

Liver failure has a number of causes that can manifest as either acute liver failure or cirrhosis. Regardless of the cause, signs and symptoms appear when there is loss of function of 80%–90% of hepatocytes. In acute liver failure, this is due to an inflammatory or necrotic process, whereas in cirrhosis this is due to the replacement of hepatocytes with fibrotic tissue.

Causes of acute liver failure include:

- Infection (viral hepatitis, Weil's disease)
- Toxins (paracetamol overdose, drug reactions)
- Budd–Chiari syndrome (liver venous outflow obstruction)
- Infiltrative diseases (Wilson's disease)
- If a patient already has established chronic liver disease, then infection, alcohol bingeing, GI bleeding and electrolyte disturbances can cause an acute-on-chronic liver failure

Cirrhosis causes include:

- Alcohol abuse (alcoholic liver disease)
- Infection (viral hepatitis B/C)
- Non-alcoholic fatty liver disease
- Drugs and toxins (methotrexate, amiodarone, isoniazid)
- Autoimmune causes: Autoimmune hepatitis, primary sclerosing cholangitis, primary biliary cirrhosis
- Vascular causes: Budd–Chiari syndrome, congestive heart failure

Metabolic causes: Wilson's disease, alpha-1-antitrypsin deficiency, sarcoidosis, haemochromatosis

CLINICAL PRESENTATION

Acute liver failure

Acute liver failure presents with sudden onset of severe illness with:

- Jaundice
- Hypoglycaemia (due to depleted glycogen stores)
- Features of decompensation: Hepatic encephalopathy (due to ↑ ammonia), haemorrhage (↓ clotting), ascites
- Patients may have hepatomegaly and signs on examination of liver failure

Cirrhosis

Often asymptomatic until there are complications of liver disease. Patients may have vague symptoms such as fatigue, nausea and weight loss. In advanced disease with derangement of liver function, symptoms include:

- Oedema (↓ albumin)
- Bruising (↓ clotting)
- Oesophageal varices + ascites + internal haemorrhoids (portal hypertension)

> **Note**: Patients with cirrhosis may not have hepatomegaly, as the liver becomes hard and smaller with fibrosis.
>
> Patients may also present with features of decompensated liver disease (see the previous section).

> **Acute alcohol withdrawal**
>
> Occurs when drinking stops suddenly:
>
> 6–12 hours: Tremor
>
> 12–24 hours: Hallucinations
>
> 24–48 hours: Withdrawal seizures
>
> 48–72 hours: Delirium tremens
>
> The Clinical Institute Withdrawal Assessment for Alcohol (CIWA-Ar) is used to assess and guide treatment.
>
> Benzodiazepines are used in acute withdrawal. B-vitamin complex can also be given.

EXAMINATION

General inspection: Jaundice, gynaecomastia, spider naevi (found in distribution of IVC), bruising.

Hand signs: Clubbing, white nails (↓ albumin), Dupuytren's contracture, palmar erythema.

Presence of asterixis (flapping tremor) suggestive of hepatic encephalopathy.

Abdominal inspection: Skin telangiectasia, oedema, ascites, caput medusa, hypogonadism.

Abdominal palpation: Hepatomegaly (not in cirrhosis), splenomegaly (from portal hypertension).

There may also be signs of the underlying cause, e.g. Kayser–Fleischer rings in Wilson's disease.

INVESTIGATIONS

Bedside: Urinalysis (exclude nephrotic syndrome as an alternative cause of low albumin).

Bloods: FBC (anaemia from occult bleeding, ↓ platelets, ↑ MCV from alcohol abuse), LFTs (↑ AST and ↑ ALT in intrahepatic damage, ↑ GGT in active alcoholics, ↑ bilirubin if jaundiced, ↓ albumin), U&Es (detection of hepatorenal syndrome), coagulation screen (check liver synthetic function, ↑ INR ↑ PT), screening for underlying cause (autoantibody screen, hepatitis serology, ceruloplasmin, ferritin, alpha-1-antitrypsin level).

Imaging: USS liver, transient elastography (if hepatitis C + or ↑ alcohol intake – used to detect cirrhosis).

Invasive: Biopsy was traditionally used to diagnose cirrhosis; however, it is no longer used due to the risk of adverse effects (e.g. bleeding). NICE recommend an upper endoscopy to check for oesophageal varices in new diagnosis of cirrhosis. If ascites is present, ascitic tap for MC + S, especially if acutely unwell, as spontaneous bacterial peritonitis may occur.

MANAGEMENT
Acute liver failure

Patients should be managed with an ABCDE approach; look for sepsis, hypoglycaemia and varices.

If the underlying cause is known (e.g. GI bleed, sepsis, paracetamol overdose) this should be treated.

Complications should be managed: **bleeding** (vitamin K, platelets, FFP, blood as needed ± endoscopy), **hypoglycaemia** (IV glucose), **infection** (antibiotics), **ascites** (fluid restriction, diuretics), **encephalopathy** (lactulose – removes nitrogen-forming organisms from bowel to ↓ ammonia levels), **malnourishment** (thiamine and folate supplementation). Vitamin B_1 should always be given prior to intravenous dextrose to minimise the risk of precipitating Wernicke–Korsakoff syndrome. Liver transplantation may be offered if patients meet the criteria listed in the following section.

Chronic
Non-pharmacological

- Education about the condition and alcohol abstinence
- Diet advice ensuring adequate nutrition and with a reduced protein intake
- Vaccinations against hepatitis A, influenza and pneumococcal infection
- Osteoporosis risk assessment (patients with cirrhosis are at an increased risk)
- Surveillance for complications:
  - Model for end-stage liver disease (MELD) score completed every 6 months for complications
  - Ultrasound ± alpha-fetoprotein every 6 months to monitor for hepatocellular carcinoma
  - Upper endoscopy every 3 years to detect oesophageal varices (Table 3.4.1)

Pharmacological

- Medications available depend on the underlying cause of cirrhosis
- If malnourished, give thiamine and folate supplementation (deficiency in thiamine can lead to Wernicke's encephalopathy – a triad of ataxia, ophthalmoplegia and confusion – that can ultimately lead to the irreversible Korsakoff syndrome [as for Wernicke's but with anterograde and retrograde amnesia])

Surgical

Liver transplantation is the curative treatment for cirrhosis.

Table 3.4.1 King's College Hospital criteria and Child–Pugh score

King's College Hospital criteria for liver transplantation		Child–Pugh score of cirrhosis and risk of variceal bleeding			
Paracetamol liver failure	**Non-paracetamol failure**		1 point	2 points	3 points
Arterial pH <7.3 after ingestion OR all from: PT > 100 s Creatinine >300 μmol/L Encephalopathy with incoherence or coma (Grade III/IV)	PT >100 s OR 3/5 from: 1. Drug-induced failure 2. Age <10 or >40 years 3. >1 week from jaundice to encephalopathy 4. PT >50 s 5. Bilirubin ≥300 μmol/L	Bilirubin (μmol/L)	<34	34–51	>51
		Albumin (g/L)	>35	28–35	<28
		PT (sec > normal)	1–3	4–6	>6
		Ascites	None	Slight	Moderate
		Encephalopathy	None	1–2	3–4

3.5 JAUNDICE

DEFINITION

Jaundice is a clinical sign describing yellow pigmentation of the skin, sclera and mucous membranes as a result of a raised plasma bilirubin. It can be caused by a number of disorders.

EPIDEMIOLOGY

The incidence of jaundice in the UK is estimated to be 56 per 100,000 people.

AETIOLOGY

Jaundice can be classified into prehepatic, intrahepatic or posthepatic (*Table 3.5.1*).

In intrahepatic jaundice, the ALT and AST are usually disproportionately elevated in comparison to the ALP and GGT, whereas in posthepatic (obstructive) jaundice, the ALP and GGT are disproportionately elevated in comparison to the ALT and AST. Isolated raised ALP and GGT can be due to a number of pathologies, such as high bone turnover and alcohol intake, respectively. Intrahepatic jaundice may also demonstrate failure of the synthetic function of the liver on LFTs (e.g. platelets and clotting).

PATHOLOGY

Bilirubin metabolism (and thus how different types of jaundice present) can be divided into three stages:

Prehepatic: Haem molecules from RBC are degraded by macrophages to bilirubin. If there is increased red cell breakdown, there is an increase in the amount of bilirubin in the body. As the bilirubin has not reached the liver, it has not been conjugated and so prehepatic jaundice has a rise in unconjugated bilirubin. The two inherited syndromes that cause prehepatic jaundice are due to deficiencies in the conjugation enzyme, leading to a rise in unconjugated bilirubin.

Intrahepatic: In the liver, bilirubin is removed from the blood by hepatocytes and conjugated. If there is breakdown of hepatocytes (due to inflammation, injury, vascular congestion or infiltration) then there is a release of conjugated bilirubin.

Posthepatic: Conjugated bilirubin has been made water soluble by hepatocytes and is transported out of the liver and into the biliary system to be stored in the gallbladder. Therefore, pathology that obstructs the biliary tree (gallstones, cancer, inflammation) causes a backlog of bilirubin that cannot be secreted into the gastrointestinal tract.

CLINICAL PRESENTATION

Patients may present with an isolated jaundice or have symptoms suggestive of underlying pathology, including abdominal pain (hepatitis/gallstones), weight loss, anorexia (pancreatic cancer – discussed in the following section).

When clerking, ask about blood transfusions, recent travel, IVDU, tattoos, sexual activity, family history, alcohol consumption and medications.

An important feature to ask about is stool and urine colour. In posthepatic jaundice, **pale stools** occur as no bilirubin makes it to the GI tract and it is therefore excreted via the urine, turning it **dark**.

> **Note**: A 2-week wait referral should be made if a patient presents with jaundice and weight loss!

EXAMINATION

When examining a patient with jaundice, look for evidence of the underlying cause:

Table 3.5.1 Classification of jaundice

	Prehepatic	Intrahepatic	Posthepatic
Bilirubin	Unconjugated	Conjugated	Conjugated
Causes	**Haemolytic anaemia** (see Section 8.1) **Gilbert's syndrome** (relative glucuronyl transferase deficiency) **Criggler–Najjar syndrome** (absolute glucuronyl transferase deficiency) **Drugs** (e.g. antimalarials)	**Hepatitis** (see Section 9.1) **Alcoholic liver disease** **Hepatocellular carcinoma** **Right heart failure** **Budd–Chiari syndrome** **Infiltrative disease** (e.g. Wilson's disease, hereditary haemochromatosis) **Drugs** (e.g. paracetamol overdose)	**Gallstones** (see Section 12.1) **Pancreatic cancer** **Pancreatitis** (see Section 12.2) **Cholangiocarcinoma** **Autoimmune** (primary biliary cirrhosis, primary sclerosing cholangitis) **Drugs** (e.g. co-amoxiclav)
LFTs	↑ Bilirubin	↑ ALT, ↑ AST, ↑ bilirubin May show ↓ platelets	↑ ALP, ↑ GGT, ↑ bilirubin

- Signs of chronic liver disease (e.g. palmar erythema, clubbing, gynaecomastia, spider naevi)
- Signs of liver failure (altered mental state, bruising, petechiae)
- Lymphadenopathy (the presence of Vichow's node could suggest pancreatic cancer)
- Abdominal masses:
  - Hepatomegaly: Alcoholic liver disease, hepatitis, hepatocellular carcinoma, metastases
  - Splenomegaly: Haematological disorders, portal hypertension secondary to liver failure
  - Palpable gallbladder: Courvoisier's sign – a palpable gallbladder in a jaundiced person is likely to be due to extra-hepatic obstruction (e.g. pancreatic cancer) and not gallstones
- Abdominal tenderness
  - Assess for Murphy's sign (see Section 12.1)
- If heart failure suspected as a cause, perform a cardiovascular examination looking for evidence of right heart failure (see Section 1.2)

INVESTIGATIONS

Bedside: Urine dipstick (if positive for bilirubin suggestive of increased levels of conjugated bilirubin).

Bloods: FBC (identify haemolysis or infection), LFTs (identify type of jaundice), U&Es (hepatorenal syndrome), clotting screen (assess liver synthetic function), amylase (if pancreatitis suspected), hepatitis serology (if suspected), autoantibody screen (anti-mitochondrial antibody raised in PBC, ANCA raised in PSC), tumour markers (CA19-9 for pancreatic, AFP for hepatocellular), serum ferritin (haemochromatosis), ceruloplasmin (Wilson's).

Imaging: USS liver (identify obstructive pathology), CT/MRI if malignancy is suspected.

Invasive: MRCP (if gallstones suspected), liver biopsy.

MANAGEMENT

Management of a patient with jaundice will depend on the underlying cause. Some of these are discussed elsewhere in this book (see section references).

Intrahepatic

Hepatocellular carcinoma: Malignant tumour of hepatocytes. Caused by viral hepatitis (persistent HBV or HCV), cirrhosis and anabolic steroids. Alpha-feto protein is the tumour marker. Treatment is resection and transplantation.

Wilson's disease: Autosomal recessive disorder with accumulation and deposition of copper in the liver and CNS. Present with liver failure or psychiatric problems. Signs include copper deposits in the skin (bronzing) and eyes (Kayser–Fleischer rings); ↑ 24-h urinary copper excretion and serum ↓ caeruloplasmin. Treatment is lifelong penicillamine, lower copper diet and potentially liver transplantation if severe disease.

Hereditary hemochromatosis: Inherited disorder of iron metabolism. Deposition of iron in organs leads to skin pigmentation, diabetes, chronic liver disease, hepatomegaly, osteoporosis, arthralgia and cardiomyopathy. Bloods show ↑ AST, ↑ ALT, ↑ ferritin, ↑ serum iron, ↓ TIBC. Treatment is with venesection.

Posthepatic

Pancreatic cancer: Classically presents late as a painless obstructive jaundice. ↑ CA19-9. Most cancers are adenocarcinomas and are too advanced for resection so are treated palliatively. If resectable, a proximal, distal or total pancreaticoduodenectomy is performed.

Primary biliary cirrhosis: Autoimmune-mediated interlobular damage causing progressive cholestasis. Often asymptomatic until ↑ ALP and ↑ IgM found on bloods. More common in women and associated with other autoimmune conditions (e.g. RA, pSS, thyroid). Majority are anti-mitochondrial antibody M2-positive. Treatment is symptomatic for pruritus (e.g. cholestyramine), diarrhoea (e.g. codeine) and osteoporosis prevention. Liver transplantation is a last resort.

Primary sclerosing cholangitis: Autoimmune condition causing inflammation and fibrosis of the bile ducts. Patients may be asymptomatic but may develop liver failure. Associated with IBD (especially UC). Blood tests show positive ANCA. At risk of developing cholangiocarcinoma. Liver transplantation is the only effective treatment.

3.6 UPPER GASTROINTESTINAL BLEED

DEFINITION

A gastrointestinal (GI) bleed is a bleed that can occur anywhere along the GI tract. It can be broadly defined as an upper GI bleed or a lower GI bleed. Upper GI bleeding occurs proximal to the ligament of Treitz, whereas lower GI bleeding occurs distally.

EPIDEMIOLOGY

Upper GI bleeding is the most common emergency managed by gastroenterologists in the UK and has an overall incidence of 50–150 per 100,000 people per year. It accounts for 5000 deaths each year in the UK.

AETIOLOGY

The causes of upper GI bleeding can be classified by their anatomical location:

Oesophageal: Oesophagitis, oesophageal varices, oesophageal cancer, Mallory–Weiss tear

Gastric: Peptic ulcer disease, gastritis, malignancy.

Duodenal: Peptic ulcer disease.

Other causes for an upper GI bleed include medications (e.g. warfarin), bleeding disorders and hereditary haemorrhagic telangiectasia (HHT).

The most common cause of an upper GI bleed is peptic ulcer disease, with duodenal ulcers being more common than gastric ulcers (around 30% and 20%, respectively).

PATHOLOGY

Specific pathologies that can present with an upper GI bleed include:

Peptic ulcer disease (PUD): Breach in the gastric/duodenal epithelium developing an ulcer. Caused by *Helicobacter pylori* infection, drugs (NSAIDs, aspirin, bisphosphonates, corticosteroids), smoking or Zollinger–Ellison syndrome (gastrinoma).

Oesophageal varices: Abnormal, dilated veins in the lower one-third of the oesophagus that occur secondary to portal hypertension, most commonly due to cirrhosis.

Oesophageal cancer: Most commonly adenocarcinomas of the lower one-third of the oesophagus because of the metaplasia caused by GORD (Barrett's oesophagus). Risk factors include GORD, obesity, smoking, alcohol.

Mallory–Weiss tear: A mucosal laceration to the epithelium of the oesophagus that occurs after repeated episodes of vomiting.

Gastric cancer: Most commonly adenocarcinomas of the stomach. Risk factors include *H. pylori* colonisation, smoking, high nitrate diet (smoked foods), blood group A. Increased risk with pernicious anaemia.

CLINICAL PRESENTATION

The two characteristic findings of upper GI bleeding are haematemesis (bright red or coffee-ground vomit) and melaena (black, tarry stool due to partly digested blood).

Patients may present acutely with these symptoms (which may lead to syncope + shock) or they may present with a chronic bleeding picture of tiredness and fatigue secondary to iron deficiency anaemia.

Other symptoms for specific conditions include dyspepsia (PUD, oesophageal cancer), dysphagia (oesophageal cancer), weight loss (oesophageal + gastric cancer), previous multiple episodes of vomiting (Mallory–Weiss tear), relationship to food (pain **worsened** by food → **gastric** ulcer [gastric acid aggravating the ulcer], pain **eased** by food → **duodenal** ulcer due to HCO_3^- secretion in preparation for digestion).

EXAMINATION

Depending on the cause and severity of the upper GI bleed, patients may be in shock (↑ HR, ↓ BP) and have tenderness to palpation of the epigastric region (oesophageal varices, peptic ulcer disease). Postural hypotension should be assessed as resting hypotension is a LATE sign of hypovolaemia.

On abdominal examination, you should look for evidence of:

- Cachexia: Indicating potential underlying malignancy
- Lymphadenopathy: In particular, Virchow's node indicates a potential gastrointestinal malignancy
- Stigmata of liver disease (e.g. palmar erythema, gynaecomastia, spider naevi) suggestive of oesophageal varices as a cause of the GI bleed

Scoring systems

For an upper GI bleed, there are two scoring systems that need to be calculated. The **Glasgow–Blatchford** score is used to identify patients at risk of needing immediate endoscopic management for their bleeding. The **Rockall** score is used to identify patients at high risk of an adverse outcome after an acute upper GI bleed.

INVESTIGATIONS

Bedside: BP, ECG, urine output.

Bloods: FBC (check Hb – may be normal in acute bleeding due to haemodilution not yet taken place), U&Es (isolated rise in urea out of proportion to creatinine suggests digested blood), LFTs (cirrhosis), cross-match, INR (check bleeding time), clotting, blood glucose.

Imaging: CXR and AXR (check for perforation from PUD).

Invasive: Endoscopy.

DIFFERENTIAL DIAGNOSIS

The most common differential diagnoses of an upper gastrointestinal bleed are duodenal ulcer (30%), gastric ulcer (20%), acute erosions or gastritis (20%),

Mallory–Weiss tear (10%), oesophageal varices (5%), oesophagitis (5%) and oesophageal cancer (<3%).

MANAGEMENT

Acute upper GI bleeding should be managed using an ABCDE approach. Unstable patients should be resuscitated and have an **endoscopy immediately**. All other patients should have an endoscopy **within 24 hours of admission**. The management options for an acute upper GI bleed fall broadly for those who are likely to have **variceal bleeding** (suggested by volume of haematemesis/critically unwell, signs/bloods of chronic liver disease) and those with **non-variceal bleeding**.

Variceal bleeding

Prior to endoscopy, patients will require prophylactic antibiotics and terlipressin (ADH analogue that reduces pressure within the portal system).

Endoscopic management options of variceal bleeding include band ligation, glue injection or thrombin injection. For uncontrolled bleeding, options include balloon tamponade or transjugular intrahepatic portosystemic shunt (TIPSS).

Ongoing management following endoscopy involves regular review and medications such as propranolol to prevent further bleeding.

Non-variceal bleeding

Proton pump inhibitors should be given pre- and postendoscopy. Endoscopic management options include mechanical clips or thermal coagulation with adrenaline.

Peptic ulcer disease

Initial management involves lifestyle management (weight loss, stop smoking, avoid food triggers) and testing the person for *Helicobacter pylori* with either a carbon-13 urea breath test or stool antigen test — **ensure the person has not taken a PPI in the past 2 weeks, or antibiotics in the past 4 weeks**.

- If the patient tests positive for *H. pylori* with a proven gastric or duodenal ulcer then start the patient on **triple 'eradication therapy'** (PPI, metronidazole, amoxicillin [or clarithromycin if penicillin-allergic]).

- If the patient tests negative for *H. pylori* with a proven gastric or duodenal ulcer, then prescribe a PPI for 4–8 weeks and review.

- Referral should be made under the 2-week wait for patients with:
  - Dysphagia/upper abdominal mass consistent with stomach cancer
  - Patients aged ≥55 years with weight loss and either upper abdominal pain, reflux or dyspepsia

- Non-urgent referrals for investigation of upper gastrointestinal cancer should be made for:
  - Patients presenting with haematemesis to primary care
  - Patients ≥55 years with treatment-resistant dyspepsia, upper abdominal pain and ↓ Hb, nausea/vomiting with weight loss, reflux, dyspepsia, upper abdominal pain or ↑ Pts

REFERENCE

National Institute for Health and Care Excellence. NICE Upper Gastrointestinal Cancer Referral Guidelines. https://cks.nice.org.uk/gastrointestinal-tract-upper-cancers-recognition-and-referral

GASTROENTEROLOGY: QUESTIONS

3.1 CROHN'S DISEASE

1. Which part of the gastrointestinal tract does Crohn's disease affect?
2. Which vitamin and nutrient deficiencies should be screened for in patients with Crohn's disease?
3. What are the extra-intestinal features of inflammatory bowel disease?

3.2 ULCERATIVE COLITIS

1. Which part of the gastrointestinal tract does ulcerative colitis (UC) affect?
2. What are the features of a severe flare of ulcerative colitis?

3.3 COELIAC DISEASE

1. What are the pathological changes in the small bowel in coeliac disease?
2. What clinical signs may you elicit in a patient with coeliac disease?
3. What are the first-line investigations for the diagnosis of coeliac disease?

3.4 LIVER FAILURE

1. Name three causes of acute liver failure.
2. What are the features of liver decompensation?
3. What are the signs of liver failure that may be elicited on examination?

3.5 JAUNDICE

1. What are the causes of prehepatic jaundice and what will the LFTs likely show?
2. What are the causes of intrahepatic jaundice and what will the LFTs likely show?
3. What are the causes of posthepatic jaundice and what will the LFTs likely show?

3.6 UPPER GI BLEED

1. Name three causes of upper GI bleeding.
2. What are the scoring systems used when a patient presents with an upper GI bleed?
3. Which medications are often given to patients with oesophageal varices prior to their endoscopy?

CHAPTER **4**

Endocrinology

4.1 TYPE 2 DIABETES MELLITUS

DEFINITION

Type 2 diabetes mellitus (T2DM) is a syndrome of chronic hyperglycaemia (persistent hyperglycaemia – HbA1c >48 mmol/mol [6.5%] or random plasma glucose >11 mmol/L) caused by a combination of insulin resistance and insulin deficiency.

EPIDEMIOLOGY

T2DM is the most common form of diabetes (90%). In the UK, 5%–10% of individuals have T2DM.

The condition classically occurs in adulthood in overweight individuals and is becoming increasingly prevalent in childhood. Asian and African ethnic groups are at a higher risk of developing T2DM.

AETIOLOGY

Multifactorial (environment + genetic): There is a 90% concordance rate among monozygotic twins and the risk of developing T2DM is 10× higher if there is a first-degree relative with the condition.

Mature onset diabetes of the young (MODY) is a rare autosomal dominant T2DM caused by a number of single gene changes.

Obesity and adipokines from adipocytes contribute to insulin resistance.

Secondary diabetes can occur from pancreatic diseases (chronic pancreatitis, pancreatic cancer, hereditary haemochromatosis, removal of pancreas), endocrine disease (Cushing's syndrome, phaeochromocytoma, acromegaly) and drugs (corticosteroids, atypical antipsychotics).

Risk factors for T2DM include obesity, lack of physical activity, a history of gestational diabetes and taking certain medications (thiazide diuretics and corticosteroids, atypical antipsychotics).

CLINICAL PRESENTATION

Patients may be asymptomatic. Typical features include thirst, polyuria, blurred vision, weight loss, recurrent infections and fatigue. May have features of the complications of T2DM (*Table 4.1.1*).

EXAMINATION

Look for features of insulin resistance (acanthosis nigricans), dyslipidaemia or a secondary cause of T2DM.

Look for features of peripheral vascular disease: Check peripheral pulses and CRT.

Look for evidence of diabetic retinopathy: Perform ophthalmoscopy.

Look for evidence of diabetic neuropathy: Perform a neurological examination.

INVESTIGATIONS

Bedside: Urinalysis (evidence of nephropathy and ACR measurement), finger prick glucose, BMI

Table 4.1.1 Complications of T2DM

Macrovascular complications	Microvascular complications
Peripheral vascular disease Intermittent claudication, arterial ulceration	**Diabetic retinopathy** Reduction in vision, increased risk of vitreous haemorrhage and maculopathy
Ischaemic heart disease Angina, myocardial infarction	**Diabetic nephropathy** Chronic kidney disease
Cerebrovascular disease Stroke, transient ischaemic attack	**Diabetic neuropathy** Peripheral neuropathy, autonomic neuropathy, Charcot's arthropathy

Examination station

A common examination station is to examine the foot of a diabetic patient. Make sure you inspect their **heels for evidence of deformity, skin condition, callus and ulcers**; also **palpate pulses** and **check CRT**. Neurologically, check **sensation, vibration sense** and **ankle jerks**. Diabetic patients commonly have a '**glove-and-stocking**' distribution to their peripheral neuropathy, with the **loss of light touch and vibration occurring first**. This is known as the '**loss of protective sensation**'.

measurement, ophthalmoscopy (evidence of retinopathy), blood pressure.

Bloods: Blood glucose, HbA1c (diagnosis/monitoring), triglycerides, cholesterol, LFTs, renal function (T2DM ↑ risk of NASH/NAFLD/cirrhosis).

Diagnosis of T2DM

If the patient is **symptomatic**:

Fasting glucose ≥7.0 mmol/L

Random glucose ≥11.1 mmol/L (or after 75 g oral glucose tolerance test)

If the patient is **asymptomatic**, the aforementioned criteria apply but must be demonstrated on **two separate occasions**.

An HbA1c of ≥6.5% (48 mmol/mol) is diagnostic of diabetes mellitus.

MANAGEMENT

Non-pharmacological

- Lifestyle management (diet, exercise, smoking cessation, reduce alcohol consumption)

Table 4.1.2 Stepwise medical management of hyperglycaemia in T2DM

Once diet and lifestyle measures optimised

If HbA1c ≥6.5% start **metformin** (unless contraindicated)

If HbA1c rises to ≥7.5% start dual therapy with either **sulfonylurea** or **DPP4-inhibitor** or **pioglitazone** or **SGLT-2i**

If HbA1c remains ≥7.5% consider starting either:

- Triple therapy with metformin, a gliptin and a sulfonylurea, or
- Triple therapy with metformin, pioglitazone and a sulfonylurea, or
- Triple therapy with metformin, pioglitazone or a sulfonylurea and an SGLT-2i
- Insulin-based therapy: Typical regimes include:
  - 1/2/3 Daily injections of combination therapies (short acting + intermediate acting)
  - Basal-bolus regime (long-acting insulin with rapid acting before meals)
- If triple therapy is ineffective or not tolerated, then a trial of a **GLP-1 mimetic (exenatide)** if the patient has a BMI >35, or if BMI <35 and would have significant occupational implications for starting insulin-based therapy

- Educate about the condition
- Offer structured group education programme (Diabetes Education for Self-Management for Ongoing and Newly Diagnosed [**DESMOND**])
- Monitor for complications (inform about annual screening for retinopathy, foot problems, nephropathy and cardiovascular risk factors)

Pharmacological

- Stepwise regime for glycaemic control (*Tables 4.1.2, 4.1.3*)
  - Lipid modification: Offer either atorvastatin 20 mg for primary prevention if QRISK2 >10% or age >85 years or atorvastatin 80 mg for secondary prevention of cardiovascular disease
- Blood pressure: ACE inhibitor is first line for all patients with diabetes diagnosed with hypertension (if African/Caribbean, prescribe concurrent diuretic or calcium channel blocker)

REFERENCE

National Institute for Health and Care Excellence. NICE Guidelines on Type 2 Diabetes. https://www.nice.org.uk/guidance/ng28

Table 4.1.3 Medications used in the management of T2DM

Biguanides	Sulphonylureas	Metaglitinides
Metformin	*Gliclazide, tolbutamide, glibenclamide*	*Repaglinide, nateglinide*
Reduce the rate of gluconeogenesis and increase insulin sensitivity	Act on beta cells to promote insulin secretion in response to glucose and other secretagogues	Insulin secretagogues
		Act via closure of K+-ATP channel in beta cells
Do not affect insulin secretion or cause hypoglycaemia or predispose to weight gain	Ineffective in patients with no remaining beta cell function	Short-acting agents that promote insulin secretion in response to meals
Side effects: Diarrhoea	Side effects: Promote weight gain, risk of hypoglycaemia	
Thiazolidinediones	**Dipeptidyl peptidase-4 inhibitors (DPP4)**	**GLP-1 agonists**
Glitazones (pioglitazone)	*Saxagliptin, sitagliptin, etc.*	*Exenatide, liraglutide*
Reduce insulin resistance by interaction with PPAR-y receptor	Enhance the incretin effect (oral glucose response >IV glucose due to GLP-1 and GIP)	Injectable long-acting analogues of GLP-1
Reduce hepatic glucose production and enhance peripheral glucose uptake	Side effects: Nausea, pancreatitis	Promote insulin release, inhibit glucagon release, reduce appetite and delay gastric emptying
Pioglitazone is the only remaining agent but has adverse effects: Fluid retention, heart failure and bladder cancer	NICE advise continuing DPP-4 inhibitor only if there is a reduction of >0.5 percentage points in HbA1c in 6 months	Major advantage is glucose control with weight reduction
		Given by subcutaneous injection before meals
		NICE advises patients to have achieved a 1% reduction in HbA1c and 3% weight loss after 6 months to justify the ongoing prescription of GLP-1 mimetics
Gliflozins	**Insulin: Mechanism of action**	**Insulin: Examples**
Dapagliflozin, canagliflozin	Promotes glucose uptake into tissues	**Rapid-acting**: Insulin aspart (Novarapid)
SGLT2 inhibitors that prevent reabsorption of glucose by the kidney tubules	Stimulates glycogen, fatty acid and protein synthesis	**Short-acting**: Insulin neutral (Actrapid/Humulin S)
	Inhibits gluconeogenesis	**Intermediate-acting**: Isophane insulin (Humulin M3)
Side effects: Urinary tract infections, weight loss	Side effects: Hypoglycaemia, weight gain	**Long-acting**: Insulin glargine (Lantus), insulin detemir (Levemir)

4.2 HYPOTHYROIDISM

DEFINITION

Hypothyroidism is the clinical picture that occurs when there is deficiency of thyroid hormone.

EPIDEMIOLOGY

Hypothyroidism is common, affecting 4/1000 people per year.

AETIOLOGY/PATHOLOGY

The causes of hypothyroidism can be divided into primary and secondary causes. The overwhelming majority of cases are primary hypothyroidism. Secondary hypothyroidism is rare and caused by ↓ TSH (hypopituitarism).

Causes of primary hypothyroidism include:

- Primary atrophic hypothyroidism: Common, lymphocytic infiltrate of the gland – **Autoimmune**
- Hashimoto's thyroiditis: Goitre due to lymphocytic and plasma cell infiltration. Occasionally can have a period of hyperthyroidism prior to hypothyroidism – **Autoimmune**
- Iodine deficiency (most common cause worldwide)
- Post-thyroidectomy or radioiodine treatment
- Drugs: Amiodarone (can cause hypothyroidism and hyperthyroidism as structurally like T_4), lithium
- Subacute thyroiditis (can also have period of hyperthyroidism prior to hypothyroidism)
- Riedel's thyroiditis: Replacement of thyroid tissue with fibrotic tissue. IgG4-related disease

CLINICAL PRESENTATION

Patients with hypothyroidism classically present with symptoms of fatigue, intolerance to cold, weight gain, constipation, amenorrhoea and depression.

EXAMINATION

Signs on examination can be remembered by the mnemonic **BRADYCARDIC**: **B**radycardia, **R**eflexes (slow), **A**taxia (cerebellar), **D**ry thin hair/skin, **Y**awning/drowsy, **C**old hands, **A**scites ± non-pitting oedema, **R**ound face, **D**efeated demeanour, **I**mmobile, **CC**F.

Steps for clinically examining the thyroid include:

Observation: Weight status, behaviour, skin changes, goitre.

Hands: Presence of other autoimmune disorders (see box), thyroid acropachy (pseudoclubbing), onycholysis,

---

Associated autoimmune conditions

- Type 1 diabetes mellitus
- Vitiligo
- Coeliac disease
- Pernicious anaemia

---

finger prick marks (diabetes), warmth, pulse rate (↓), myoexedema.

Face: Round (puffy with periorbital oedema), hair thinning, loss of lateral eyebrow hair. Look from the side of the patient for the presence of enophthalmos.

Neck:

- Front: Inspect for scars, presence of a neck lump, asymmetry. Palpate the carotid pulse and assess the tracheal position. Percuss down the upper part of the sternum to assess for dullness indicating a retrosternal goitre. Auscultate for bruits over the thyroid
- Back: Palpate for the thyroid gland. If palpable, describe characteristics (size, shape, texture, tender); palpate the anterior and posterior triangles of the neck and check for any cervical lymphadenopathy

Manoeuvres:

- Goitre: Ask the patient to take a sip of water and swallow. A goitre will move upwards on swallowing. If a goitre is present, check for dysphonia (enlargement of the goitre can affect the recurrent laryngeal nerve)
- Thyroglossal cyst: Ask the patient to stick their tongue out. A thyroglossal cyst will move upwards on protrusion

Peripheral thyroid examination: Check biceps reflex (slow-relaxing), assess for proximal myopathy (ask the patient to stand from sitting without using their arms) and carpel tunnel syndrome.

INVESTIGATIONS

Bedside: ECG (bradycardia).

Bloods: TFTs (↑ TSH, ↓ T3), autoantibodies (thyroid peroxidase), FBC (anaemia), HbA1c (associated diabetes), lipids.

Imaging: USS scan thyroid (if lump).

DIFFERENTIAL DIAGNOSIS

The differential diagnosis for symptoms and signs similar to hypothyroidism according to NICE include sick euthyroid syndrome, other autoimmune conditions (coeliac, diabetes, adrenal insufficiency, pernicious anaemia), haematological conditions (anaemia, myeloma), anxiety and depression, chronic fatigue syndrome.

MANAGEMENT

Non-pharmacological

- Educate about the condition
- Consider screening for other autoimmune conditions associated with hypothyroidism
- Conduct a cardiovascular risk assessment

Pharmacological

- Levothyroxine (LT4) daily
- Review the patient every 3–4 weeks after initiation and adjust the dose according to clinical and biochemical parameters, aiming for resolution of symptoms and signs of hypothyroidism and a normal serum TSH. Look for signs of side effects (see box)

Side effects of thyroxine treatment

- Hyperthyroidism (overtreatment)
- Reduced bone mineral density
- Worsening angina
- Atrial fibrillation

Interactions of levothyroxine

- Iron (give 2 hours apart from levothyroxine as iron ↓ absorption of levothyroxine)
- Calcium carbonate (↓ levothyroxine absorption)
- COCP, antiepileptics and rifampicin can increase LT4 requirements

Refer to an endocrinologist if the patient:

- Has a goitre, nodule or structural change in the thyroid gland
- Is suspected of having associated endocrine disease (e.g. adrenal failure)
- Has adverse effects from levothyroxine treatment
- Is female and planning a pregnancy
- Has preexisting cardiac disease
- Has persistently elevated TSH despite adequate treatment

4.3 HYPERTHYROIDISM

DEFINITION

Hyperthyroidism is the clinical picture that occurs when there is an excess of thyroid hormone.

EPIDEMIOLOGY

The majority of hyperthyroidism is caused by Graves' disease, which occurs in 0.5% of the population.

It affects women more than men (9:1).

AETIOLOGY/PATHOLOGY

Graves' disease is an autoimmune condition that accounts for the majority of cases worldwide.

It is a **triad of goitre, eye signs and thyrotoxicosis**. Circulating IgG autoantibodies bind to and activate G-protein-coupled thyrotropin receptors, which causes enlargement of the thyroid gland and increases thyroid hormone secretion. Associated with type 1 DM, vitiligo and Addison's.

Other causes of hyperthyroidism include:

- Toxic multinodular goitre: Nodules that secrete thyroid hormone, treated with radioiodine/surgery.
- Toxic adenoma: Solitary nodule producing thyroid hormone. Appears 'hot' on isotope scan. Treated with radioiodine.
- Ectopic thyroid tissue (e.g. from choriocarcinoma, ovarian teratoma).
- Exogenous thyroid (diet, excess levothyroxine).
- Subacute (de Quervain's) thyroiditis: Postviral hyperthyroidism with a painful goitre. Investigations show a raised ESR and low isotope uptake on scan. Treated with NSAIDs.
- Iatrogenic: Amiodarone, lithium.
- Postpartum thyroiditis: Occurs in 7% of women a year after giving birth.

CLINICAL PRESENTATION

The symptoms of hyperthyroidism can be remembered by the mnemonic **SWEAT²I²NG²**: **S**weating, **W**eight loss, **E**motional lability, **A**ppetite increased, **T**remor/**T**achycardia, **I**ntolerance of heat/irregular menstruation/**I**rritability, **N**ervousness, **G**oitre/**G**I problems (diarrhoea).

EXAMINATION

Signs that may be elicited on examination include clammy hands, tachycardia, fine tremor, palmar erythema, lid lag, goitre and thyroid bruit. Graves' disease is associated with pretibial myxoedema, thyroid acropachy and eye signs (see box).

Steps for clinically examining the thyroid include:

> ### Eye signs in Graves' disease
> - Lid lag, lid retraction
> - Periorbital oedema
> - Exophthalmos
> - Exposure keratopathy
> - Ophthalmoplegia

Observation: Weight status, behaviour, skin changes, goitre.

Hands: Presence of other autoimmune disorders (see box), thyroid acropachy (pseudoclubbing), onycholysis, finger prick marks (diabetes), warmth, pulse rate ($\uparrow$).

Face: Hair thinning. Look from the side of the patient to look for the presence of eye signs. Assess for lid lag by holding your finger superiorly and asking the patient to follow it with their eyes whilst keeping their head still. Move your finger down whilst observing the patient's upper eyelids. If lid lag is present, the upper eyelids will be observed lagging behind the eye's downward movement.

Neck:

- Front: Inspect for scars, presence of a neck lump, asymmetry. Palpate the carotid pulse and assess the tracheal position. Percuss down the upper part of the sternum to assess for dullness indicating a retrosternal goitre. Auscultate for bruits over the thyroid.
- Back: Palpate for the thyroid gland. If palpable, describe characteristics (size, shape, texture, tender). Palpate the anterior and posterior triangles of the neck and check for any cervical lymphadenopathy.

Manoeuvres:

- Goitre: Ask the patient to take a sip of water and swallow. A goitre will move upwards on swallowing. If a goitre is present, check for dysphonia (enlargement of the goitre can affect the recurrent laryngeal nerve).
- Thyroglossal cyst: Ask the patient to stick their tongue out. A thyroglossal cyst will move upwards on protrusion.

Peripheral thyroid examination: Check biceps reflex (brisk), assess for proximal myopathy (ask the patient to stand from sitting without using their arms), pretibial myxoedema.

INVESTIGATIONS

Bedside: ECG (tachycardia/AF).

Bloods: TFTs ($\downarrow$ TSH, $\downarrow\uparrow$ T3), autoantibodies (anti-TSH receptor), FBC (anaemia), HbA1c (associated diabetes), lipids.

Imaging: USS scan thyroid (if lump).

> **Complications of hyperthyroidism**
> - Cardiovascular (heart failure, angina, AF)
> - Osteoporosis
> - Ophthalmopathy

MANAGEMENT
Non-pharmacological
- Education about the condition
- Monitor for complications

Pharmacological
- Symptomatic relief with a beta-blocker (propranolol) to provide relief of adrenergic symptoms
- Antithyroid medication (two regimes):
  - Titration with carbimazole
  - Block and replace with carbimazole and levothyroxine (↓ risk of iatrogenic hypothyroidism)
- Radioiodine can be used but most become hypothyroid post-treatment. CI in pregnancy

Surgical
- Indications for thyroidectomy include:
  - Intolerance to medication
  - Failure of medication
  - Preference of surgical treatment
  - Large goitre
- Complications of surgery include:
  - Bleeding (the thyroid has a dual blood supply from the superior thyroid artery (originates from the common carotid artery) and the inferior thyroid artery (originates from the subclavian artery – see Figure 4.3.1)
  - Recurrent laryngeal nerve injury (the nerve is in close proximity to the thyroid and injury can lead to a hoarse voice)
  - Hypocalcaemia (due to hypoparathyroidism if the parathyroid glands are damaged)
  - Hypothyroidism
  - Recurrent hyperthyroidism

> **Causes of a goitre**
> - *Diffuse*: Graves', physiological (pregnancy/puberty), Hashimoto's thyroiditis, subacute thyroiditis (painful)
> - *Nodular*: Multinodular goitre, tumours (benign/malignant), adenoma
> - Also consider infiltrative diseases such as sarcoidosis. TB may also infiltrate the thyroid gland.

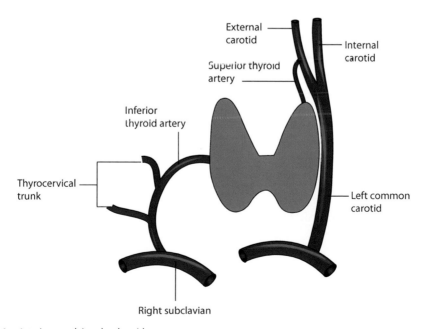

Figure 4.3.1 Arteries supplying the thyroid.

4.4 CUSHING'S SYNDROME

DEFINITION

Cushing's syndrome refers to the clinical state resulting from persistently and inappropriately elevated levels of glucocorticoid and the loss of the feedback mechanism of the hypothalamic–pituitary–adrenal (HPA) axis.

EPIDEMIOLOGY

Cushing's syndrome can occur for a variety of reasons. Corticosteroids (e.g. prednisolone) are prescribed frequently and these are the chief cause of Cushing's syndrome. Endogenous causes (see next) are rare.

AETIOLOGY

Cases of Cushing's syndrome can be divided into those that have a ↑ ACTH or a ↓ ACTH.

ACTH-dependent causes (↑ ACTH)

- Cushing's disease (pituitary adenoma)
- Ectopic secretion from tumour (small-cell lung cancer)

ACTH-independent causes (↓ ACTH)

- Iatrogenic: Steroids (most common)
- Adrenal adenoma
- Adrenal carcinoma

PATHOLOGY

Cortisol release is usually controlled via the HPA axis. Corticotropin-releasing factor (CRF) is released from the hypothalamus and stimulates ACTH secretion from the anterior pituitary gland. ACTH then stimulates cortisol and androgen production in the adrenal cortex. Therefore, ACTH-dependent causes of Cushing's are secreting ACTH to stimulate the adrenal cortex to secrete cortisol, hence ACTH is raised. In ACTH-independent causes, cortisol is being released by the adrenal gland (or iatrogenic steroids) themselves, so the level of ACTH is reduced due to the normal feedback mechanism of the HPA.

The excess tissue exposure to cortisol leads to dysfunction of carbohydrate, lipid and protein metabolism. Cortisol stimulates the release of glucose into the blood stream, leading to **hyperglycaemia**. The disorder of lipid metabolism causes **fat deposition**. The loss of collagen due to the protein dysfunction leads to **purple striae**. Cortisol also inhibits osteoblast function and encourages bone resorption, leading to **osteoporosis**.

Disruption of sex hormones in the adrenal cortex may lead to **amenorrhoea** and **erectile dysfunction**. Disruption of mineralocorticoid function from the adrenal cortex may lead to **fluid retention** and **hypertension**. Patients may also have recurrent infections due to a suppressed immune system.

Excessive corticosteroids can suppress prostaglandin secretion leading to gastrointestinal ulcers.

CLINICAL PRESENTATION

The presenting features of Cushing's syndrome include ↑ weight, proximal myopathy, mood change (depression, insomnia, psychosis), sex hormone dysfunction (amenorrhoea, erectile dysfunction), recurrent infections, fracture and GI bleed (from peptic ulcers).

EXAMINATION

A patient with Cushing's syndrome may exhibit the following features that can be identified on systemic examination:

- Hands: Bruising, thinning of the skin
- Arms: Measure blood pressure (hypertension), check for interscapular fat pad
- Face: Note any mooning of the face
- Abdomen: Presence of striae
- Legs: Assess for proximal myopathy (stand up from chair without using their arms)

Following your examination, you can palpate the spine (assessing for tenderness to look for a vertebral crush fracture), offer to check blood glucose and examine for a visual field defect (due to Cushing's disease).

Importantly, check for evidence of any condition the patient may have for which they may have to take corticosteroids (RA, asthma, COPD etc.).

INVESTIGATIONS

Bedside: BP (hypertension).

Bloods: FBC (check WCC due to immunosuppression), blood glucose (↑), U&Es (↓ K+).

Imaging: CT adrenals, pituitary MRI.

Special investigations

The investigations performed when Cushing's syndrome is suspected can be divided into confirmation and localisation tests.

Confirmation tests

- Overnight dexamethasone suppression test
    - 1 mg dexamethasone given at night and cortisol is measured in the morning
    - In a normal state, the cortisol level will be reduced due to negative feedback
    - If the cortisol remains high despite dexamethasone, this indicates there has been no suppression of the HPA axis, which confirms Cushing's syndrome
- 24-hr urinary free cortisol is an alternative

Localisation tests

- Plasma ACTH
  - If low: CT adrenals (look for adrenal tumour)
  - If high: Perform high-dose dexamethasone suppression test (8 mg):
    - If cortisol is low: Cushing's disease
    - If cortisol is high: Look for ectopic ACTH source (e.g. small-cell lung cancer, thyroid)

MANAGEMENT

Depends on the cause:

- Iatrogenic: Discontinue the steroids if possible
- Adrenal adenoma or carcinoma: Removal of adrenal gland and radiotherapy if carcinoma
- Cushing's disease: Transsphenoidal removal of adenoma
- Ectopic ACTH: Removal of causative tumour if no metastases

4.5 ADRENAL GLAND DISORDERS

ADDISON'S DISEASE (PRIMARY ADRENAL INSUFFICIENCY)

Definition

Addison's disease is caused by destruction of the adrenal cortex. This leads to the reduced production of the products from each layer of the adrenal cortex (see box). This leads to a reduction in the production of glucocorticoids, mineralocorticoids and adrenal androgens.

Epidemiology

Addison's disease is rare in clinical practice, with less than <10,000 people in the UK having the condition. In the developed world, it is most commonly caused by an autoimmune process, where it may coexist with other autoimmune conditions (such as T1DM). Worldwide, TB is the most common cause.

Layers of the adrenal cortex

GFR

Glomerulosa (produces aldosterone)

Fasciculata (produces cortisol)

Reticularis (produces precursor androgens (e.g. DHEA)

Aetiology

Autoimmune, TB, metastases (e.g. bronchial carcinoma), meningococcal septicaemia (Waterhouse–Friderichsen syndrome), HIV, antiphospholipid syndrome.

Pathology

Addison's disease is the primary insufficiency of the adrenal gland, meaning that the lack of production caused by a problem within the adrenal gland is resulting in the insufficiency (see box). Because the rest of the hypothalamic–pituitary–adrenal (HPA) axis is working correctly, an excess of ACTH is produced by negative feedback, which forms the basis behind the short Synacthen® test (see box). ACTH is itself a product of a larger precursor protein, POMC, which also produces melanocyte-stimulating hormone (MSH). The increase in ACTH production causes an increase in MSH, leading to pigmentation, a hallmark of Addison's disease.

Types of adrenal insufficiency

Primary: Addison's disease

Secondary: Pituitary disorders (e.g. tumours, irradiation, infiltration)

Tertiary: Stopping exogenous steroids

Short Synacthen test

Synthetic ACTH is given, ideally in the morning Synacthen 250 μg is used.

Cortisol is measured at baseline (pre-Synacthen), 30 and 60 minutes.

In a normal patient, cortisol should rise in response to ACTH (usually >450 nmol/L).

A failure to rise (less than double baseline) indicates primary adrenal insufficiency (Addison's disease).

Clinical Presentation

Symptoms of Addison's disease are often non-specific (fatigue, anorexia, mood changes) but classically patients present with postural hypotension (due to the lack of aldosterone) and hyperpigmentation (due to ↑ MSH production). Patients may also present in an acute adrenal crisis, which may be precipitated by intercurrent infection, stress or steroid withdrawal. Features include hypovolaemic shock, acute abdominal pain, vomiting and fever.

Examination

In a stable patient, perform a sitting and standing blood pressure to check for a postural drop. Examine the hands and mouth looking for evidence of hyperpigmentation (prominent in the palmar creases and buccal mucosa). Examine for the presence of other concurrent autoimmune diseases such as T1DM, hypothyroidism and vitiligo. You should also examine for evidence of the underlying causes (e.g. TB).

Investigations

Bedside: BP, finger prick glucose.

Bloods: FBC (infection markers), U&Es ($\downarrow$ Na$^+$, $\uparrow$ K$^+$), blood glucose (concurrent T1DM), B$_{12}$/folate (concurrent pernicious anaemia), adrenal antibodies. Short Synacthen test is the definitive investigation.

Imaging: CXR (TB), adrenal CT.

Differential Diagnosis

NICE suggests a differential diagnosis of an acute abdomen, depression, gastroenteritis, eating disorders, T1DM and chronic fatigue syndrome in patients presenting with symptoms similar to Addison's disease.

Management

Acute adrenal insufficiency

If acute adrenal insufficiency (Addisonian crisis) is suspected, measure cortisol, blood glucose and U&Es.

Resuscitate the patient with IV fluids if shocked and give replacement hydrocortisone immediately, without waiting for results of cortisol.

Correct any electrolyte abnormalities (e.g. ↑ K$^+$) and hypoglycaemia.

Investigate for precipitating factor (e.g. blood cultures for sepsis).

Get help from endocrinology to investigate the underlying cause and for long-term management.

Chronic disease
Non-pharmacological
Educate the patient about the condition and warn of the 'sick-day rules' (see box). Provide cortisol for IM administration and teach patient/partner how to administer.

Pharmacological
Treat the underlying cause. Give replacement corticosteroids (prednisolone) and mineralocorticoids (fludrocortisone) if needed. Dehydroepiandrosterone (DHEA) may be prescribed if androgen replacement needed.

Steroid use

Need to carry a steroid card and a medic-alert bracelet

Never miss a dose

Sick-day rules

Doubling of steroid dose for febrile illness

Admission for parenteral steroids if vomiting, diarrhoea, severe illness

---

REFERENCE
National Institute for Health and Care Excellence. NICE Guidelines on Addison's Disease. https://cks.nice.org.uk/addisons-disease

PRIMARY HYPERALDOSTERONISM
Definition
Primary hyperaldosteronism is the clinical state produced by excess production of the mineralocorticoid aldosterone, which is produced in the zona glomerulosa of the adrenal cortex.

Epidemiology
Primary hyperaldosteronism is now cited as the most common cause of secondary hypertension, with an estimated 5%–10% prevalence in individuals diagnosed with hypertension.

Aetiology
The principal causes of primary hyperaldosteronism are bilateral idiopathic adrenal hyperplasia and adrenal adenoma (Conn's syndrome). Rarer causes include an adrenal carcinoma.

Pathology
Aldosterone acts on the principal cells in the distal tubule and collecting duct of the kidney. It upregulates and activates basolateral Na$^+$/K$^+$ pumps, which creates a concentration gradient that results in reabsorption of sodium and secretion of potassium leading to **hypernatraemia** (and thus **hypertension**) and **hypokalaemia**. Aldosterone also stimulates H$^+$ secretion via H$^+$/ATPase in intercalated cells, leading to a **metabolic alkalosis**.

Clinical Presentation
Patients are often asymptomatic and may be found to have incidental hypertension. Patients may develop symptoms of hypokalaemia (see Section 7.4).

EXAMINATION
Patients may have no findings but may demonstrate hypertension on BP measurement. Other signs include dehydration (from hypernatraemia) or signs from hypokalaemia (see Section 7.4).

Investigations
Bedside: BP, urinalysis.

Bloods: U&Es (↑ Na$^+$, ↓ K$^+$), serum aldosterone levels (↑), serum renin levels (↓).

Imaging: CT abdomen (used to differentiate between adrenal hyperplasia and adrenal adenoma).

Management
Non-pharmacological
Education about the condition.

Pharmacological
Spironolactone (an aldosterone antagonist) can be given for bilateral idiopathic adrenal hyperplasia.

Surgical
Adrenalectomy for adrenal adenoma.

ENDOCRINOLOGY: QUESTIONS

4.1 TYPE 2 DIABETES MELLITUS

1. Name three risk factors for the development of type 2 diabetes mellitus.
2. What are the macrovascular and microvascular complications of type 2 diabetes mellitus?
3. How can type 2 diabetes mellitus be diagnosed?
4. What are the mechanisms of action of the drugs metformin, gliclazide and dapagliflozin?

4.2 HYPOTHYROIDISM

1. What signs may be elicited on examination in a patient with hypothyroidism?
2. Name three causes of hypothyroidism.
3. Which autoimmune conditions are associated with autoimmune hypothyroidism?

4.3 HYPERTHYROIDISM

1. Which antibodies may be present in Graves' disease?

2. What are the medical management options for hyperthyroidism?
3. What are the complications of hyperthyroidism?

4.4 CUSHING'S SYNDROME

1. What are the ACTH-dependent causes of Cushing's syndrome?
2. What are the ACTH-independent causes of Cushing's syndrome?
3. What tests can be performed to confirm the presence of Cushing's syndrome?

4.5 ADRENAL GLAND DISORDERS

1. What are the layers of the adrenal cortex and what do they produce?
2. What is the definitive diagnostic test for Addison's disease?
3. What are the electrolyte abnormalities seen in primary hyperaldosteronism?

Rheumatology

5.1 RHEUMATOID ARTHRITIS

DEFINITION

Rheumatoid arthritis (RA) is an autoimmune disease that causes persistent synovitis resulting in a chronic symmetrical polyarthritis and systemic inflammation.

EPIDEMIOLOGY

Around 1% of the population have RA. It is more common in women (3:1) and typically presents at 30–50 years.

AETIOLOGY

Multifactorial aetiology:

- Familial: Increased incidence in first-degree relatives
- Genetic: Associated with HLA-DR4 and HLA-DRB-1

PATHOLOGY

Inflammation of the synovium leading to the formation of a **pannus** (abnormal granulation tissue) from an influx of inflammatory cells. Cells in the granulation tissue contract causing destruction and fusion of the joint.

CLINICAL PRESENTATION

Symptoms suggestive of synovitis:

- Pain: Worse at rest and during periods of inactivity
- Swelling: Around the joint – feels boggy when palpating
- Stiffness: Lasts >30 minutes in the morning and after periods of inactivity

Systemic features: Fatigue, fever, weight loss.

Involvement of other body systems (see box on extra-articular manifestations).

Extra-articular manifestations of RA

The extra-articular manifestations of RA can be remembered by the mnemonic **CROCS** (which is easy to remember as RA patients have pain in their feet!)

Cardiac involvement: Pericarditis, endocarditis, ischaemic heart disease

Respiratory involvement: Pleural effusions, interstitial lung disease, Caplan's syndrome

Ocular involvement: Keratoconjunctivitis sicca, episcleritis, scleritis

Circulation: Anaemia of chronic disease, vasculitis, amyloidosis, Felty's syndrome

Soft-tissue: Rheumatoid nodules, carpal tunnel syndrome, atlanto-axial subluxation, palmar erythema, osteoporosis

Depression is also common in chronic disease such as RA.

Types of RA

Chronic persistent: Typical form follows a relapsing and remitting pattern.

Palindromic: Involves monoarticular attacks lasting up to 48 hours, may move from one joint to another.

Remitting: Active for a number of years but then remits.

Seronegative: Negative rheumatoid factor (RF), has a better long-term prognosis.

Rapidly progressive: Rapid joint damage and disability, high incidence of complications.

EXAMINATION

Examine the hands dorsally first, inspecting for evidence of:

- Symmetrical joint involvement
- Swelling of MCP and PIP joints
- Ulnar deviation (and swelling of the ulnar styloid – known as a piano key deformity)
- Any palmar subluxation of the MCP joints
- **Active synovitis**: Hot, swollen joints that are painful to touch

Ask the patient to turn their hands over and inspect the palms for evidence of:

- Thenar eminence wasting (due to carpal tunnel syndrome)
- Palmar erythema
- Boutonnière or swan neck deformity

Palpate the joints and squeeze the MCP joints (warn the patient first as this may elicit pain) and test movements. Importantly, test the function of their hands – ask to see how they hold a pen/penny.

Check for rheumatoid nodules on the extensor surfaces (commonly elbows).

Examine for evidence of psoriatic patches to help narrow down your differential (always look behind the ears!).

INVESTIGATIONS

Bloods: FBC – normochromic, normocytic anaemia (anaemia of chronic disease), thrombocytosis (active RA), CRP/ESR – raised, serology – rheumatoid factor (+ in 70%), anti-cyclic citrullinated peptide (anti-CCP) (more specific).

Imaging: Joint x-ray looking for: **LESS**: **L**oss of joint space, **E**rosions, **S**oft tissue swelling, **S**oft bones (peri-articular osteopenia).

If looking for extra-articular manifestations/differentials:

- U&Es: RA can affect renal function (amyloid deposits) and most treatments need baseline function
- LFTs: Elevations of ALP and GGT are common in active RA

- CXR: Lung involvement is common
- Antinuclear antibodies (ANA): May suggest connective tissue disease, but ANA is positive in up to 30% of people with RA

DIFFERENTIAL DIAGNOSIS

The differential diagnosis for RA includes psoriatic arthritis, reactive arthritis, connective tissue disease and osteoarthritis (with inflammation).

MANAGEMENT

When patients first present to their GP they are offered analgesia (paracetamol +/− codeine) and rheumatology referral. If pain is not controlled, then an NSAID (or coxib) + PPI can be used. Urgent review is needed (<2 weeks) if small joints (hands/feet) are affected, if >1 joint affected or delay in presentation of 3 months.

Chronic disease
Non-pharmacological

- Patient education (e.g. versus arthritis resources) about disease
- Advise to stop smoking
- Physiotherapy and occupational therapy input

- Dietary changes (RA patients at higher risk of IHD – Mediterranean diet recommended)

Pharmacological

- Monotherapy of a conventional DMARD: Methotrexate is typically first line. See Table 5.1.1 for examples of conventional DMARDs
- Biologics (e.g. etanercept/adalimumab/infliximab/tocilizumab) can be used in the treatment of RA in combination with methotrexate, or as monotherapy (except infliximab) if there is:
  - Persistent high level of disease activity (>5.1 DAS28 score on two occasions) **AND**
  - Failed treatment on combination of DMARDs
- JAK/STAT inhibitors (baricitinib/tofacitinib) can be considered with the aforementioned criteria
- For management of flares:
  - Use NSAIDs + paracetamol/codeine for symptom control of flares
  - If severe flare, oral or injected corticosteroids can be given

Surgical

Surgery can be used for patients who do not respond to optimal non-surgical treatment and should be referred for a surgical opinion.

Table 5.1.1 Examples of DMARDs used in RA

DMARD	MoA	Side effects	Monitoring
Methotrexate	Folate antagonist	Neutropenia Renal impairment GI disturbance Abnormal liver biochemistry Pulmonary fibrosis	Baseline CXR, FBC, U&Es, LFT FBC, U&E, LFT every 2 weeks for 6 weeks Then every 2–3 months
Hydroxychloroquine	Antimalarial	Photosensitivity Retinopathy (1 in 2000)	Baseline FBC, U&Es, LFT, visual acuity Annual review by optometrist
Leflunomide	Pyrimidine synthesis inhibitor	Diarrhoea Neutropenia Alopecia Hypertension	Baseline FBC, U&Es, LFT, creatinine, weight, BP FBC, LFT every 6 months, BP each visit

5.2 SERONEGATIVE SPONDYLOARTHROPATHIES

DEFINITION

The seronegative spondyloarthropathies are a group of conditions that share a number of characteristics:

- Affect the spine and peripheral joints
- Negative rheumatoid factor
- Associated with HLA-B27
- Uveitis

The seronegative spondyloarthropathies include psoriatic arthritis, ankylosing spondylitis and reactive arthritis. Enteropathic arthritis is considered another seronegative spondyloarthropathy, which is associated with inflammatory bowel disease.

PSORIATIC ARTHROPATHY

Definition

Psoriatic arthritis (PA) is an inflammatory arthritis that occurs in 10%–15% of patients who suffer from psoriasis, usually between the ages of 30–50 years, affecting men and women equally.

Clinical Presentation

Psoriatic arthropathy presents before/after onset of psoriasis. The most common type is a peripheral symmetrical polyarthritis (similar to rheumatoid arthritis), which affects 30%–40% of sufferers. Other types include:

- Asymmetrical oligoarthritis usually affecting the small joints of the hands and feet
- Sacroiliitis
- DIP joint disease
- Arthritis mutilans (severely deformed fingers/hands)

The joint pain described is typically inflammatory sounding, e.g. 'morning stiffness which eases with activity'. Patients may complain of joint pain or swelling or pain around the ligament attachments to bone (enthesitis).

Examination

There may be evidence of nail signs (e.g. onycholysis, subungual hyperkeratosis) and psoriatic patches (see Section 10.2). The type of psoriatic arthropathy will depend on which joints are affected on examination (e.g. symmetrical vs. asymmetrical etc.).

Investigations

Blood tests reveal a negative rheumatoid factor and may show↑ ESR. IgA is raised in two-thirds of sufferers. Imaging in the form of x-ray or MRI may reveal erosions such as joint subluxation, enthesitis or a pencil-in-cup deformity.

A bedside Psoriatic Arthritis Response Criteria (PsARC) should be calculated to monitor disease activity – this involves examination of the number of tender or swollen joints, completing a global pain assessment (out of 10) and a global health assessment (out of 5) from both the doctor and patient.

Management

Non-pharmacological

Education about the condition and optimisation of cardiac risk factors.

Pharmacological

Analgesia and NSAIDs for joint pain. DMARDs in the form of methotrexate and sulfasalazine slow the development of joint damage, and agents such as ciclosporin can control both the arthritis and skin lesions. Anti-TNF therapies (e.g. etanercept) are recommended if a patient has peripheral arthritis with three or more tender and swollen joints where there has been an inadequate response to at least two DMARDs. Biologics (e.g. secukinumab) can also be used and are recommended if a patient does not respond to a TNF-alpha inhibitor after 12 weeks.

ANKYLOSING SPONDYLITIS

Definition

Ankylosing spondylitis (AS) is a chronic inflammatory rheumatic disease that typically affects men (3:1) in early adulthood (20–30 years).

Clinical Presentation

AS typically affects more men than women (3:1) and causes inflammatory lower back pain (stiffness and pain worse at night that eases on getting up, back pain that eases with activity, no improvement with rest). AS also causes sacroiliitis (inflammation of the sacroiliac joints) and enthesitis, the latter of which leads to ankylosis (fusion).

AS can also cause an asymmetrical peripheral arthritis and fatigue. AS has a number of extra-articular manifestations that can be remembered as the 5 **A**s: **A**nterior uveitis, **A**ortic incompetence, **A**myloidosis, **A**pical lung fibrosis, **A**V block.

Examination

Schober's test is used as a sign of reduced forward flexion in AS (a test of lumbar flexion). The examiner finds the L5 vertebrae and marks 5 cm below and 10 cm above this point. The patient is then asked to touch their toes while keeping their knees straight. If the distance between the two points does not increase by at least 5 cm, this is a sign of lumbar flexion restriction.

Investigations

Bedside: A disease assessment tool should be used to assess patients in clinic. A common tool is the BAS-DAI score (http://basdai.com/) that asks questions about the severity of fatigue, axial joint pain, peripheral joint pain, joint swelling and discomfort resolving from waking up on a scale of 0 to 10. The questionnaire also asks how long a patient's morning stiffness lasts before resolving. It is a helpful indicator of severe disease and can be used to assess patients who benefit from anti-TNF therapy.

Blood tests: FBC, CRP and ESR to look for evidence of inflammation. An HLA-B27 test is not a reliable tool for diagnosis but can be helpful in differentiating between ankylosing spondylitis and other cases of undifferentiated axial spondyloarthropathy.

Imaging: X-ray of the spine and sacroiliac joints, ultrasound and MRI provide evidence for diagnosis. Common radiological findings for a patient with AS include sacroiliitis, spinal fusion and syndesmophytes (new bony formations in the intervertebral joint ligaments). A late radiological finding is a 'bamboo-spine' on x-ray.

Management
Non-pharmacological
Education about the condition, morning exercise regime, multidisciplinary team involvement, regular assessments for osteoporosis.

Pharmacological
NSAIDs for joint pain (unless contraindicated), corticosteroid injections. Anti-TNF therapies (such as etanercept) can be used in patients who cannot tolerate, or if their disease does not respond to, NSAIDs. Response to Anti-TNF therapy is assessed by the BAS-DAI score. Surgery may be indicated in the form of joint replacement or spinal straightening.

REACTIVE ARTHRITIS
Definition
Reactive arthritis is an arthritis that occurs following an infection where the organism cannot be recovered from the joint. It classically occurs following either an STI or gastroenteritis but can occur following any infection. Reactive arthritis following STI acquisition is more common in men (10:1).

Clinical Presentation
Reactive arthritis typically causes an asymmetrical lower limb oligoarthritis around 4 weeks following the infection. Other symptoms include urethritis, conjunctivitis, circinate balanitis (painless vesicles on the prepuce) and keratoderma blennorrhagia (waxy rash on the soles of feet). The majority of patients have a single attack that settles, but some may be left with a relapsing arthritis. A cohort of patients may have an initial resolution of the joint pain but may suffer recurrences.

Investigations
Investigations are used to exclude the differential diagnosis.

Bloods: Serology for detection of typically organisms such as *Chlamydia* can be used.

Invasive: Joint aspiration can rule out septic arthritis.

Management
Non-pharmacological
Education about the condition and advice about hygiene/sexual activity if appropriate. Pharmacological: Symptomatic management in the form of NSAIDs/analgesics/corticosteroid injections. Chronic disease may require DMARDs.

5.3 SYSTEMIC LUPUS ERYTHEMATOSUS

DEFINITION

Systemic lupus erythematosus (SLE) is a systemic inflammatory autoimmune disease where autoantibodies are made against a variety of autoantigens. Immune system dysfunction leads to deposition of immune complexes in various organs (e.g. kidneys) leading to systemic symptoms.

EPIDEMIOLOGY

SLE affects 0.2% of the UK population, more commonly in women (9:1) and in people of Afro-Caribbean origin.

When SLE occurs in men, it is commonly associated with Klinefelter's syndrome (47, XXY).

AETIOLOGY

The cause of SLE is unknown but is thought to be multifactorial:

- Genetic:
  - A number of genes have been linked to the development of SLE (>20)
  - Higher concordance rate in monozygotic twins compared to dizygotic
- Environmental:
  - Epstein–Barr virus has been suggested as a trigger for SLE
  - Some drugs cause a form of SLE (drug-induced lupus), e.g. hydralazine, procainamide, penicillamine and isoniazid

PATHOLOGY

In SLE there is a malfunction in apoptosis. Usually during apoptosis, self-antigens are contained within the fragments of the cell (blebs) and are hidden from the immune system. In SLE, there is inefficient removal of blebs by phagocytosis and self-antigens are ultimately presented to antigen-presenting cells in the lymphoid tissue, stimulating production of antibodies against these self-antigens. These autoantibodies then damage host tissue by type II and III hypersensitivity and inflammatory reactions.

CLINICAL PRESENTATION

SLE is a multisystem disorder and can present with a number of different features. Classically, the presenting patient is a young female (premenopausal) presenting with non-specific symptoms (fatigue, malaise and fever) with arthralgia and a skin rash (classically a malar rash, which spares the nasolabial folds, or a photosensitive rash across the face and chest).

The clinical manifestations of SLE are summarised in *Table 5.3.1*.

EXAMINATION

As SLE is a multisystem disease, there can be a variety of signs to find on examination. If you have a patient

Table 5.3.1 Manifestations of SLE

System	Manifestations
Joints	Peripheral small joint arthritis (may present to similar to RA) in 90% of patients
Skin	Malar (butterfly) rash in 30% of patients
	Photosensitive rash
	Discoid lupus (raised erythematous patches with keratotic scales and scarring)
	Livedo reticularis
	Raynaud's phenomenon
	Alopecia
Nervous system	Seizures/psychosis in the absence of explainable cause/trigger
	Mood disorder and anxiety can occur
	Migraine is common
Respiratory	Pleuritis causing chest pain or pleural effusions causing dyspnoea
	Can also manifest as a fibrosing alveolitis causing a restrictive lung defect
Kidneys	Proteinuria
	Lupus nephritis is a severe manifestation of SLE and can cause end-stage renal failure
	The most common manifestation is diffuse proliferative glomerulonephritis
Cardiovascular	Pericarditis, myocarditis, pericardial effusions, vasculitis
	A sterile form of endocarditis can also occur (Libman–Sacks endocarditis)
Gastroenterology	Oral and aphthous ulceration
Haematology	Haemolytic anaemia, leucopenia, lymphopenia or thrombocytopenia can occur
	Antiphospholipid syndrome occurs in 20%–30% (see box)

with SLE as a long case in your examinations, then your medical school may ask you to perform a particular examination (e.g. upper limb musculoskeletal examination) due to time pressures. Otherwise if you can perform a systemic examination look for:

Hands: Examine the small joints of the hand and look for evidence of vasculitis or Raynaud's phenomenon.

Upper limb: Perform a BP reading.

Head and neck: Look for evidence of hair loss, malar rash, discoid lupus and photosensitivity.

Chest: Perform a respiratory examination looking for evidence of a pleural effusion and a cardiovascular examination looking for evidence of a pericardial rub suggestive of pericarditis.

Abdomen: Look for evidence of a renal transplant scar (from lupus nephritis).

INVESTIGATIONS

May vary depending on the systems affected.

Bedside: Urinalysis (looking for proteinuria), blood pressure (↑ due to lupus nephritis), ECG (pericarditis).

Bloods: Immunology (see box), FBC (detect haematological disturbance – see *Table 5.3.1*), U&Es (lupus nephritis), inflammatory markers (↑ ESR but normal CRP is common), vitamin D (deficiency is common and can manifest in similar non-specific symptoms).

Imaging: USS kidneys, DEXA scan (osteoporosis risk), CXR (if respiratory/cardiovascular symptoms).

Invasive: Skin/renal biopsy (can be used if uncertainty about diagnosis).

Immunology in SLE

- 99% are anti-nuclear antibody (ANA) positive.
- Anti-dsDNA is highly specific for SLE (99%) but less sensitive than ANA (70%) and can be used for disease monitoring.
- Anti-Smith is the **most** specific antibody for SLE but has a low sensitivity (30%).
- Complement (C3, C4) are low during active disease (they are consumed during complex deposition).

MANAGEMENT
Acute disease

Severe SLE flares are characterised by haemolytic anaemia, lupus nephritis, pericarditis or CNS disease. They require specialist management and immunosuppression (usually cyclophosphamide and prednisolone).

Chronic disease
Non-pharmacological

- Avoid triggers (e.g. sun exposure) and use high-factor sunblock to prevent rashes
- Topical steroids can be used for skin rashes

Antiphospholipid syndrome

- Occurs in 20%–30% of SLE patients
- Disorder of venous + arterial thrombosis
- Causes: Coagulation defect, thrombocytopenia, recurrent miscarriages/ischaemic stroke and livedo reticularis
- Investigations:
  - Anticardiolipin test
  - Lupus anticoagulant
  - Anti-B2-glycoprotein test
- Treatment:
  - Aspirin or warfarin
  - Seek advice if pregnant

Other autoantibodies in rheumatology

Rheumatoid arthritis: RF, anti-CCP

Polymyositis: Anti-Jo-1

Limited systemic sclerosis: Anti-centromere

Diffuse systemic sclerosis: Anti-Scl70

Primary Sjögren's syndrome: Anti-Ro, La

Mixed connective tissue disease: Anti-RNP

Drug-induced lupus: Anti-histone

- Assess risk for osteoporosis and cardiovascular disease (as patients are at ↑ risk)

Pharmacological

- Joint pain can be managed with NSAIDs and DMARD therapy (e.g. hydroxychloroquine)
- Biologics can be used but have not shown the dramatic effect as they have in other diseases; belimumab is the current recommended add-on therapy in SLE if dsDNA is positive and complement levels are low

Surgical

- Renal transplant may be required in severe lupus nephritis.

5.4 GOUT

DEFINITION

Gout is an inflammatory crystal arthropathy caused by the deposition of monosodium urate monohydrate in the synovium of joints. It is caused by a chronic hyperuricaemia (uric acid >450 μmol/L) although not all raised urate levels cause gout!

EPIDEMIOLOGY

Gout is the most common inflammatory arthritis with an estimated prevalence of 2%–3% in the UK. It is more common in men and typically occurs in adulthood with an increasing prevalence with age.

AETIOLOGY

Uric acid is produced as a breakdown product of purine metabolism and produced by the enzyme xanthine oxidase. Excess purine ingestion from diets contain large amounts of saturated fat and fructose, which contribute to increased levels. Purines are also released during cell death.

PATHOLOGY

Hyperuricaemia is caused by either **impaired excretion** or **overproduction** of uric acid. Most commonly, the cause of gout is idiopathic (90%) due to impaired excretion of uric acid.

Risk factors for developing gout include obesity, alcohol intake, drugs that increase plasma urate levels (thiazide diuretics, aspirin), hypertension, renal failure/impairment, diabetes mellitus, hyperlipidaemia, vascular disease, lead intoxication and conditions that cause overproduction of uric acid such as malignancy, myeloproliferative disorders and Lesch–Nyhan syndrome.

CLINICAL PRESENTATION

Most commonly, there is an **asymptomatic period** of hyperuricaemia prior to an **acute** presentation with an **acute monoarthritis**, most commonly the **first metatarsophalangeal (MTP) joint**. Other joints that are commonly affected include the ankle, wrist and knee. Attacks may be precipitated by alcohol, food, dehydration or starting a diuretic.

Following an attack there may be intervals where patients are asymptomatic before having another attack. Prolonged hyperuricaemia may result in chronic tophaceous gout where patients have tophaceous nodules.

EXAMINATION

The affected joint may be erythematous, swollen and painful to move. If a patient has chronic tophaceous gout, they may have white deposits (tophi) in their skin and around joints. They commonly occur on the ear, fingers and Achilles tendon.

INVESTIGATIONS

Gout is often a clinical diagnosis and NICE recommends that no initial investigations are required when managing people with gout-like symptoms.

Bedside: Urinalysis (check renal function).

Bloods: Renal profile (check renal function), FBC (check for haematological disorders), serum uric acid (measured 4–6 weeks after an acute attack of gout to confirm hyperuricaemia because serum uric acid levels often fall during an attack of gout). Blood cholesterol and blood glucose may be appropriate as patients with gout are at higher risk of hyperlipidaemia and diabetes.

Imaging: Joint x-ray to look for chondrocalcinosis or to rule out other acute pathology.

Invasive: Joint fluid microscopy and culture (can be used to confirm the diagnosis of gout or rule out septic arthritis; aspiration shows the presence of **negatively birefringent needle-shaped crystals**).

DIFFERENTIAL DIAGNOSIS

The differential diagnosis for an acute gouty monoarthritis includes non-urate crystal-induced arthropathy such as **pseudogout** or **hydroxyapatite** deposition, septic arthritis, osteoarthritis, psoriatic arthritis, reactive arthritis, rheumatoid arthritis, seronegative spondyloarthropathy and haemochromatosis.

Table 5.4.1 presents the differences between gout and pseudogout.

Table 5.4.1 Comparing gout with pseudogout

	Gout	Pseudogout
Crystals	Monosodium urate	Calcium pyrophosphate
More common in	Men	Women
Causes	Idiopathic (90%) → under-excretion of MSU rarer Renal failure Lead intoxication	'Metabolic' Hyperparathyroidism Hypothyroidism Wilson's Haemochromatosis
Clinical features	Acute pain (1st MTP/wrist/hand) Tophi if chronic	Acute pain (knee/shoulder)
Arthrocentesis	Negative needle crystals	Positive rhomboid crystals
Management	Flare control: NSAIDs/colchicine ULT: Allopurinol	NSAIDs, corticosteroids, DMARDs

Table 5.4.2 Medications used in gout

Drug	Mechanism of action	Used as	Side effects
Allopurinol	Xanthine oxidase inhibitor	Urate-lowering therapy	Rash (withdraw therapy if occurs)
Febuxostat	Xanthine oxidase inhibitor	Urate-lowering therapy	Deranged LFTs
Canakinumab	Interleukin-1 inhibitor	Acute flare management	Immunosuppression
Lesinurad	Urate transporter inhibitor	Urate-lowering therapy	Rise in serum creatinine

Remember that **P**seudogout has **P**ositive birefringent crystals.

MANAGEMENT
Acute disease
- Analgesia in the form of an **NSAID** (such as diclofenac, indomethacin or naproxen) until 24–48 hours after the attack has resolved
  - If NSAIDs are contraindicated or not tolerated, prescribe oral **colchicine**
  - If NSAIDs and colchicine are contraindicated or not tolerated, give systemic corticosteroids
  - Canakinumab (IL-1 inhibitor) can also be considered instead of corticosteroids
- Gastroprotection: Co-prescribe a **PPI** (such as omeprazole) while using NSAIDs if there is a risk of peptic ulceration
- **Follow-up the patient in 4–6 weeks** and assess the following:
  - Risk factors: Measure BP, glucose, renal function and lipid profile
  - Optimise management of underlying conditions such as hypertension and diabetes
  - Provide lifestyle advice on obesity, diet, alcohol consumption and exercise
  - Measure the patient's serum uric acid level in 4–6 weeks after the acute attack

- Assess the need for prophylaxis – it is now recommended that allopurinol is initiated after the first attack of gout. NSAIDs/colchicine cover should be used when starting allopurinol

Chronic disease
Non-pharmacological
Lifestyle advice (stop smoking, diet advice, exercise, reduce alcohol consumption, aim for ideal body weight, avoid dehydration).

Pharmacological
- The British Society for Rheumatology now advocates allopurinol after the first attack of gout
- Check the patient's renal function prior to starting allopurinol and recheck every 12 months
- Febuxostat is another xanthine oxidase inhibitor that can be used instead of allopurinol if allopurinol does not adequately reduce uric acid levels (see *Table 5.4.2*)

REFERENCES
National Institute for Health and Care Excellence. NICE Guidelines Gout. https://cks.nice.org.uk/gout

British Society for Rheumatology Gout Guidelines. https://academic.oup.com/rheumatology/article/56/7/e1/3855179

5.5 OSTEOPOROSIS

DEFINITION

Osteoporosis is a disease characterised by reduced bone mass and structural deterioration of bone tissue with an increase in bone fragility and susceptibility to fracture.

EPIDEMIOLOGY

Osteoporosis is common after the age of 50 years and is more prevalent in women than men (3:1). The prevalence of osteoporosis increases with age, with approximately 2% at the age of 50 to almost 50% at 80 years of age.

AETIOLOGY

Osteoporosis may be primary or secondary to another condition or medication. Risk factors for developing osteoporosis can be remembered by the mnemonic **SH^{2}ATTERED^2**: **S**teroid use, **H**yperthyroidism/**H**yperparathyroidism, **A**lcohol and tobacco use, **T**hin (BMI <18.5), **T**estosterone ↓, **E**arly menopause, **R**enal or liver failure, **E**rosive bone disease (e.g. myeloma, RA), **D**ietary Ca^{2+} ↓/**D**iabetes.

Medications that may worsen osteoporosis include corticosteroids, SSRIs, PPIs and aromatase inhibitors.

PATHOLOGY

There are a number of regulatory systems that contribute to bone remodelling (RANK/RANKL/OPG, PTH, vitamin D, oestrogen, interleukins). When there is an issue with one or more of these systems, osteoporosis can occur. The classic example of osteoporosis occurs in postmenopausal women, where there is oestrogen deficiency. The lack of oestrogen causes an overexpression of RANKL, whose increased activity overrides the osteoclast-inhibitory effect of OPG. Therefore, a lack of oestrogen leads to increased osteoclast activity.

CLINICAL PRESENTATION

Osteoporosis is often asymptomatic until a fragility fracture occurs. When trabecular bone is affected (in the vertebrae) these can cause vertebral crush fractures, which lead to a loss of height and potentially back pain.

NICE recommends excluding any non-osteoporotic causes of a fragility fracture when clerking a patient.

Non-osteoporotic causes of fragility fracture include:

- Metastatic bone disease: Suggested by bone pain and history of cancer and raised inflammatory markers
- Multiple myeloma: Suggested by bone pain, anaemia, hypercalcaemia and renal failure (see Section 8.2)
- Osteomalacia: Suggested by bone pain, muscle pain and proximal muscle weakness
- Paget's disease of bone: Suggested by bone pain and deformity (enlargement of pelvis/spine/skull)

EXAMINATION

There are no signs on examination specific to osteoporosis, so a clinical examination should focus on seeking a secondary cause of osteoporosis.

INVESTIGATIONS

(Mainly to exclude secondary causes.)

Bedside: Urinary Bence–Jones protein (myeloma), fecal calprotectin (inflammatory bowel disease).

Bloods: FBC (infection), U&Es (renal failure), LFTs (hepatic failure), bone profile (normal or ↑ Ca^{2+}, ALP), inflammatory markers (↑ in RA/myeloma), TFTs (hyperthyroidism), PTH (hyperparathyroidism), serum testosterone (men), vitamin D levels, tissue transglutaminase (coeliac disease), amylase (pancreatitis), blood glucose (diabetes), immunoglobulins.

Imaging: **DEXA scan** (see Interpretation), x-ray.

MANAGEMENT

Non-pharmacological

- Educate about the condition
- Stop smoking and reduce alcohol intake
- Optimise BMI
- Encourage regular exercise and a balanced diet

Pharmacological

- Treat the underlying cause (if a secondary cause found)
- If bone protection medication is recommended (either by a risk-scoring tool or DEXA scan), prescribe a **bisphosphonate** (such as alendronate or risdronate) (see box)
- Other medications may also be used as protection against osteoporosis. These include:
  - Raloxifene (selective oestrogen receptor modulator): ↑ BMD in spine and fever but ↑ DVT risk
  - Denosumab (monoclonal antibody against RANKL given as injection every 6 months)
  - Teriparatide (recombinant form of PTH)
- If a patient's calcium intake is adequate but at risk of a lack of sunlight, prescribe vitamin D
- If a patient's calcium intake is inadequate, prescribe a combination of vitamin D and calcium
- If a patient has a premature menopause, consider prescribing hormone replacement therapy (HRT)

Surgical

If a patient has suffered a fragility fracture, this may require orthopaedic intervention (e.g. fractured neck of femur).

PREVENTING FRACTURES: NICE GUIDELINES

Due to the high number of fragility fractures that occur each year, NICE produced a guideline recommending who to assess for osteoporosis. They advise using a clinical prediction tool, such as FRAX or Q-Fracture in:

- All women ≥65 years
- All men ≥75 years
- Younger patients if they have risk factors, such as:
  - Previous fragility fracture
  - History of falls
  - Family history of hip fracture
  - A condition causing a secondary osteoporosis
  - Low BMI (<18.5)
  - Smoking
  - Alcohol intake >14 week for women or >21 units per week for men

Both tools generally divide patients into three categories:

- Reassure and give lifestyle advice
- Consider treatment/offer DEXA scan
- Offer bone protection treatment

INTERPRETING A DEXA SCAN RESULT

The key thing to remember about a DEXA scan result is the T-score. T-scores are determined by measuring bone mineral density at the hip.

- Normal T-score is −1.0 or higher
- T-score between −1.0 and −2.5 indicates osteopenia
- T-score of >−2.5 indicates osteoporosis

REFERENCE

National Institute for Health and Care Excellence. NICE Guidelines Osteoporosis. https://cks.nice.org.uk/osteoporosis-prevention-of-fragility-fractures

---

Bisphosphonates

Bind to hydroxyapatite to inhibit osteoclast function.

Education

Patients must only take oral bisphosphonates on an empty stomach at least 30 minutes before food with a glass of water.

Oral bisphosphonates are taken once weekly.

Be aware for the signs of side effects.

Side effects

Upper GI symptoms (dyspepsia, reflux).

Atypical fracture (e.g. groin).

Osteonecrosis of the jaw (patients need a dental check-up prior to treatment).

RHEUMATOLOGY: QUESTIONS

5.1 RHEUMATOID ARTHRITIS

1. Name three extra-articular manifestations of rheumatoid arthritis.
2. What medications can be used in the treatment of rheumatoid arthritis?
3. What are the side effects of methotrexate?

5.2 SERONEGATIVE SPONDYLOARTHROPATHIES

1. What features do the seronegative spondyloarthropathies share?

Psoriatic arthritis

1. What is the most common form of psoriatic arthritis?
2. What are the treatment options for psoriatic arthritis?

Ankylosing spondylitis

1. What is the clinical test for reduced lumbar flexion in ankylosing spondylitis?
2. What are the extra-articular manifestations of ankylosing spondylitis?

Reactive arthritis

1. What are the extra-articular signs and symptoms of reactive arthritis?
2. What is the classic triad of symptoms in reactive arthritis?

5.3 SYSTEMIC LUPUS ERYTHEMATOSUS

1. Name three organs SLE can affect and the manifestations from its involvement.
2. Which medications can cause drug-induced lupus?
3. What management options are available for treating SLE?

5.4 GOUT

1. Name three risk factors for the development of gout.
2. How should an acute attack of gout be managed and what medications can be used?
3. How do the crystals of gout differ from those that cause pseudogout?

5.5 OSTEOPOROSIS

1. Name three risk factors for osteoporosis.
2. Other than osteoporosis, what can cause a fragility fracture?
3. What pharmacological therapies can be used to treat osteoporosis?

CHAPTER **6**

Neurology

6.1 STROKE AND TRANSIENT ISCHAEMIC ATTACK

DEFINITION

Stroke refers to a syndrome of rapid onset focal or global neurological disturbance from a vascular origin (infarction/bleeding) that lasts >24 hours. A transient ischaemic attack (TIA) is an episode of transient neurological dysfunction (lasts <24 hours) caused by focal ischaemia without evidence of infarction.

EPIDEMIOLOGY

Stroke is the fourth largest single cause of mortality in the UK, with a rising incidence. There are more than 100,000 strokes per year in the UK. Around 2000 people per year have a first episode of TIA. One in 12 people (8%) will have a full stroke within a week of having a TIA.

AETIOLOGY/PATHOLOGY

The majority of strokes are ischaemic (85%) compared to haemorrhagic (15%). The most common causes of a stroke include **small vessel occlusion** (due to a **thrombus**), **emboli** (carotid/cardiac [AF/endocarditis/MI]) and CNS **haemorrhage** (aneurysm rupture, anticoagulation). TIAs are most commonly caused by emboli that may be carotid or cardiac in origin.

Risk factors for stroke and TIA include:

● Lifestyle factors (modifiable): Smoking, alcohol/drug misuse, physical inactivity and poor diet
● Previous cardiovascular disease: Hypertension, atrial fibrillation, carotid artery disease, infective endocarditis, valvular heart disease, congestive cardiac failure
● Other factors: Age, hyperlipidaemia, DM, CKD, COCP, OSA, hypercoagulable disorders

CLINICAL PRESENTATION

Stroke and TIAs present with a sudden onset of neurological deficits and may vary depending on the causative mechanism and the area of the brain affected. Focal neurological defects may include:

● Unilateral weakness/sensory loss
● Speech problems (e.g. dysphasia)
● Gait difficulties (e.g. ataxia)
● Vertigo (usually with other symptoms)
● Sudden transient loss of vision in one eye (amaurosis fugax)
● Homonymous hemianopia
● Cranial nerve defects

The symptoms caused by a TIA typically resolve within 1–2 hours but may last up to 24 hours. TIA can only be diagnosed once symptoms have resolved. If a patient has ongoing neurological symptoms of suspected vascular origin, they should be treated as a stroke.

EXAMINATION

Examination of the acute stroke/TIA patient should include a full neurological assessment, including cranial nerves. Identifying the deficits can help to confirm the diagnosis and localise the lesion. When examining the patient, it is important to assess their GCS and look for signs of a head injury. Do not miss isolated dysphasia in a patient who presents as 'confused'.

INVESTIGATIONS

Bedside: BP (↑), ECG (AF).

Bloods: Blood glucose (exclude hypoglycaemia), lipids (↑), inflammatory markers (↑ ESR in vasculitis), FBC (may show polycythaemia), blood cultures (if IE suspected).

Imaging: CT or MRI brain scan, echocardiogram (valvular lesions), CXR (enlarged left atrium).

Additionally, carotid artery ultrasound should be considered in patients with anterior circulation TIA or non-disabling stroke if the patient is willing for potential surgical intervention (carotid endarterectomy).

DIFFERENTIAL DIAGNOSIS

The most important differential diagnosis is hypoglycaemia as this can be reversed in an acute presentation.

Other differentials include head injury, subdural haemorrhage, intracranial tumours, hemiplegic migraine, post-seizure (Todd's paresis), CNS infection (e.g. toxoplasmosis, abscess, herpes encephalitis).

Oxford–Bamford Classification

Total anterior circulation syndrome (TACS)

All three of the following: (1) Unilateral weakness (and/or sensory deficit) of the face/arm/leg, (2) homonymous hemianopia, (3) higher cerebral dysfunction (e.g. dysphasia, visuospatial disorder).

Partial anterior circulation syndrome (PACS)

Any two of the following: (1) Unilateral weakness (and/or sensory deficit) of the face/arm/leg, (2) homonymous hemianopia, (3) higher cerebral dysfunction (e.g. dysphasia, visuospatial disorder), OR isolated higher cortical deficit OR isolated motor or sensory deficit of the face/arm/leg.

Posterior circulation infarct (POCI)

Any of the following: Contralateral homonymous hemianopia OR cerebellar signs OR brainstem signs (e.g. quadriplegia, gaze/visual disturbance).

Lacunar infarct (LACI)

Either a pure motor OR a pure sensory stroke OR sensorimotor symptoms in at least two from the face/arm/leg.

With four absent features: (1) No higher cortical dysfunction (cortex not affected), (2) no homonymous hemianopia (lesion not near optic radiation), (3) no drowsiness, (4) no brainstem signs.

MANAGEMENT

Acute stroke

- Use an ABCDE approach to ensure the patient's airway is supported and their observations are kept in a normal range. Do not treat ↑ BP acutely in ischaemic stroke as this may compromise circulation, but urgent BP lowering to a target of <140 mmHg systolic should be considered for haemorrhagic stroke.
- Brain imaging (usually a CT scan) is required promptly to identify a stroke as haemorrhagic or ischaemic in nature.
- Once a haemorrhagic stroke has been excluded, aspirin 300 mg should be given unless the patient is being considered for hyperacute treatment. Hyperacute treatment for ischaemic stroke includes thrombolysis and thrombectomy. These should be considered in patients who present within 4.5 hours of the onset of symptoms. Thrombectomy may be possible beyond this time window but is most effective when started early after symptom onset.

CHRONIC DISEASE

Non-pharmacological

- Stroke rehabilitation: Physiotherapy, occupational therapy, SALT, mood and cognitive screening
- Education about the condition, optimising modifiable risk factors (e.g. smoking/alcohol/weight/diet)
- Patients must not drive for at least 1 month following a stroke. If they have visual symptoms or ongoing physical symptoms after 1 month they should inform the DVLA
- Treatment of the complications of stroke (bowel/bladder problems, spasticity)

Pharmacological secondary prevention

- **Antiplatelet** therapy (if no AF) with clopidogrel or **anticoagulation** (if AF present) with warfarin/NOAC
- Control medical risk factors (hypertension, hyperlipidaemia, T2DM, obstructive sleep apnoea)

Surgical

- A carotid endarterectomy may be considered for patients with anterior circulation/TIA or non-disabling stroke if stenosis is >50% (NASCET criteria) on the same side as the TIA/stroke

TIA ASSESSMENT AND MANAGEMENT

If a patient has had a suspected TIA in the last week:

- Give 300 mg aspirin immediately (provided there is no contraindication such as bleeding disorder, allergy, or if already taking regular low dose aspirin)
- Arrange urgent assessment (<24 hours) by a stroke specialist

If a patient has had a suspected TIA that occurred more than 1 week previously:

- Arrange assessment by a stroke specialist within 7 days
- Assess for arrhythmias such as atrial fibrillation

Secondary prevention measures following a TIA are the same for stroke and involve initiating antiplatelet or anticoagulation therapy and optimising modifiable risk factors (e.g. treatment of hypertension/T2DM etc.).

REFERENCE

National Institute for Health and Care Excellence. NICE Guidelines Stroke and TIA. https://cks.nice.org.uk/stroke-and-tia

6.2 PARKINSON'S DISEASE

DEFINITION
Parkinson's disease (PD) is a chronic, progressive neurodegenerative disease resulting from the degeneration of dopaminergic neurons in the substantia nigra.

EPIDEMIOLOGY
PD is a common condition in patients >65 years of age, with a prevalence of 1%.

AETIOLOGY/PATHOLOGY
The loss of dopaminergic neurons in the substantia nigra can occur for a number of reasons resulting in parkinsonism (see box). When there is no causative condition found, idiopathic parkinsonism is termed PD.

CLINICAL PRESENTATION
The classical features of PD can be remembered by the mnemonic **TRAP**: **T**remor (present at rest), **R**igidity (↑ tone – with superimposed tremor leads to cogwheel rigidity), **A**kinesia (or bradykinesia), **P**ostural instability (without other cause).

The symptoms of PD are **asymmetrical** (used to differentiate from drug-induced parkinsonism where the symptoms are usually bilateral). Non-motor features of PD include depression (50%), dementia, rapid eye movement (REM) behaviour sleep disorder (acting out of dreams due to loss of muscle atonia during REM sleep), visual hallucinations, mild urinary frequency and urgency.

EXAMINATION
- Inspection: Expressionless face; slow blinking of the eyes; drooling.
- Hands and arms: Resting tremor (described as pill-rolling) that can be emphasised by distraction; rigidity (↑ tone) including cogwheeling at the wrist; ask the patient to use their thumb to touch each of their fingers to elicit bradykinesia.
- Face: Assess eye movements to determine any impairment in vertical gaze (a feature of PSP); assess their speech, looking for slow, monotonous speech; assess for the presence of a glabellar tap

by tapping the forehead of the patient between their eyebrows. A positive test is demonstrated by continued blinking upon tapping of the forehead (normally blinking should cease after several taps).

- Functional status: Assess a patient's handwriting looking for micrographia, ask them to pick something up/undo a button or shoelace; assess gait for:
  - Reduced arm swing (occurs early)
  - Hesitancy
  - Shuffling
  - Stooped posture
  - Hurrying (festination)

Ideally, perform a sitting and standing BP measurement (looking for postural hypotension that is a feature of MSA and PD), check for cerebellar signs (a feature of MSA) and examine the drug chart (looking for causes of drug-induced parkinsonism).

INVESTIGATIONS
PD is a clinical diagnosis and investigations are primarily used to exclude other causes of parkinsonism (e.g. Wilson's disease).

MANAGEMENT
Parkinson's disease is a progressive condition so patients with a suspected diagnosis of PD should be referred to a neurologist to initiate management.

Chronic disease
Non-pharmacological
- Multidisciplinary team involvement: Neurologist, PD nurse, physiotherapist, occupational therapist, social worker, speech and language therapy, GP and care staff
- Educate about the condition to the patient and their family and also instruct to not suddenly stop any anti-parkinsonian medication, as this can precipitate acute akinesia or neuroleptic malignant syndrome
- Patients are required to inform the DVLA about their condition

Pharmacological
- NICE Guidelines suggest the following medical management for PD (*Table 6.2.1*):
  - If motor symptoms are affecting quality of life, levodopa should be started
  - If motor symptoms are not affecting quality of life, a drug such as a dopamine agonist, a monoamine oxidase B inhibitor or levodopa can be started
  - Other medications include amantadine, COMT inhibitors and antimuscarinics
  - Advanced therapies such as duodopa and apomorphine can be used in later stages

---

Causes of parkinsonism

Idiopathic PD

Cerebrovascular disease (vascular parkinsonism)

Drug-induced (prochlorperazine, metoclopramide, antipsychotics)

Metabolic diseases (Wilson's)

Parkinson's-plus syndromes (progressive nuclear palsy [PSP], multiple systems atrophy [MSA], corticobasal degeneration [CBD])

Lewy-body dementia

Table 6.2.1   Medications used in Parkinson's disease

Medication	Examples	Mechanism of action	Side effects
Levodopa	Madopar or Sinemet Given in combination with a decarboxylase inhibitor (e.g. carbidopa) to prevent peripheral metabolism of levodopa to dopamine	Replaces the deficient dopamine in neurons in substantia nigra	Dyskinesia Palpitations Drowsiness Hypotension
Dopamine receptor agonists	Pramipexole Ropinerole	Agonist on D2 receptors	Impulse control disorders Hallucinations Hypotension
Monoamine oxidase B inhibitors	Selegiline	Inhibits the breakdown of dopamine	Hypertensive crisis Sleeplessness Dry mouth Increase levodopa and its side effects
Amantadine	–	Not fully understood but thought to increase dopamine release	Dizziness Falls Dry mouth
COMT inhibitors	Entacapone Tolcapone	Inhibits COMT enzyme that breaks down dopamine	Diarrhoea Visual hallucinations Dyskinesias

- Fludrocortisone or midodrine (an alpha-1 agonist) can be used if orthostatic hypotension requires treatment

Surgical

- Deep brain stimulation can be used as a treatment option in certain individuals with PD.

REFERENCE

National Institute for Health and Care Excellence. NICE Guidelines, Parkinson's Disease. https://cks.nice.org.uk/parkinsons-disease

6.3 EPILEPSY

DEFINITION

Epilepsy is the tendency for recurrent spontaneous, intermittent, abnormal electrical activity in the brain resulting in a transient disturbance in consciousness, behaviour, emotion, motor function or sensation. For a diagnosis of epilepsy, a patient must have at least two unprovoked seizures occurring >24 hours apart or a single seizure and an overwhelming chance that they will have a second – such as in the context of a tumour or tuberous sclerosis.

EPIDEMIOLOGY

There are approximately 32,000 new diagnoses of epilepsy each year in the UK. Epilepsy most commonly starts in childhood or in patients >60 years old and is much more common in patients with a learning disability.

AETIOLOGY

The majority of patients (2/3) with epilepsy have no identifiable cause (idiopathic). The most common identifiable causes of epilepsy include cerebrovascular disease, tumour and acquired brain injury. Other causes include hypoxic birth injury, meningitis/encephalitis, tuberous sclerosis, autoimmune causes, foetal or rare genetic syndromes.

PATHOLOGY

Mechanisms of pathology inducing epileptic seizures include increased neuronal connectivity, increased excitatory neurotransmission (↑ glutamate) or failure of inhibitory neurotransmission (↓ GABA).

CLINICAL PRESENTATION

There are a number of types of epileptic seizures that can be differentiated depending on whether they affect one cerebral hemisphere (focal) or both (generalised) at onset.

- Focal seizures (2/3 of patients with a focal seizure will develop a **secondary generalised seizure** – known as a focal seizure leading to a bilateral tonic–clonic seizure):
  - Focal seizures without impaired awareness:
    - Focal sensory seizure (sensory symptoms only)
    - Focal motor seizure
  - Focal seizure with impaired awareness (formerly complex partial seizures):
    - Focal sensory seizure: Most commonly arise from the temporal lobe causing a variety of symptoms including déjà vu/ jamais vu (familiarity/unfamiliarity), olfactory hallucinations, micropsia/macropsia (objects look little/large)
    - Focal motor seizure: These may lead to temporary paralysis (Todd's), which can cause confusion with a stroke

- Generalised seizures:
  - Absence seizures: First occur in childhood, with loss of awareness and vacant expression for <10 s and immediate recovery, can occur multiple times a day
  - Tonic–clonic seizures: Loss of consciousness with limb stiffening + jerking, initial stiff phase
  - Myoclonic seizures: Sudden muscle jerking (no loss of awareness with isolated jerks)
  - Atonic seizures: Sudden collapse with loss of muscle tone

Post-ictal confusion and headache are common following most seizure types.

When taking a history from a patient with suspected seizures you should assess for any seizure triggers (e.g. sleep deprivation, alcohol), comorbid conditions (cerebrovascular disease), symptoms of an aura (sensory focal seizure symptoms) or any features suggesting a different reason for a seizure (see differential diagnosis below). An independent eyewitness account is essential if possible; video of seizures is a boon.

EXAMINATION

The examination of a patient with epilepsy is often normal unless the patient is having a seizure or has signs of the underlying cause (e.g. limb weakness/visual field defect following a stroke). NICE recommend performing a full cardiac, neurological and mental state examination for all patients with suspected epilepsy. A seizure may be the first sign of a tumour.

INVESTIGATIONS

Bedside: ECG (arrhythmias such as heart block causing a loss of consciousness), blood pressure (lying and standing), EEG.

Bloods: FBC (anaemia), U&Es (uraemic encephalopathy), LFTs (hepatic encephalopathy), blood glucose (hypoglycaemia), bone profile (hypercalcaemia).

Imaging: CT/MRI head.

Table 6.3.1 Differentiation of non-epileptic and epileptic seizures

Feature	Non-epileptic	Epileptic
>5 minutes duration	Common	Rare
Eyes and mouth closed and resisting attempted eye opening	Common	Rare
Visible bite mark on the side of the tongue	Rare	Occasional
Respiration	Often fast	Ceases
Grunting sounds	Occasional	Common

DIFFERENTIAL DIAGNOSIS

Patients may have a seizure for a number of different reasons including fever (febrile convulsions), alcohol and drug withdrawal, hypoxia, uraemic/hepatic encephalopathy, hypoglycaemia or functional (non-epileptic) seizures (see box). Seizures are commonly mistaken for syncopal episodes (and vice versa) so it important to get a good history.

MANAGEMENT

Acute (tonic–clonic seizures)

- Protect patients having a tonic–clonic seizure from injury to the head or body by cushioning their head and removing any hazardous objects nearby. When the seizure stops, check their airway and place them into the recovery position.

- If the convulsive seizure lasts >5 minutes, or if they have had more than three seizures in an hour, in addition to the above measures manage the seizure with a benzodiazepine (such as buccal midazolam, IV lorazepam or rectal diazepam).

- Seizures lasting ≥5 minutes, or recurrent seizures without regaining consciousness lasting ≥5 minutes, are termed status epilepticus and require urgent hospital management using an ABCDE approach:
  - Give IV lorazepam, followed by another dose if no response <2 minutes
  - Open and maintain the airway and give 100% oxygen + suction (if required)
  - Gain IV access and take bloods for U&Es, FBC, glucose, calcium, toxicology screen, anticonvulsant levels
  - Correct hypotension/glucose if indicated; give thiamine if alcoholism/malnourishment is suspected
  - Give levetiracetam or phenytoin infusion if seizures continue, with ECG and BP monitoring
  - Call ICU when infusion starts – status epilepticus is a medical emergency and 'time is brain'

Chronic disease

Non-pharmacological

- Multidisciplinary team input (neurologist, epilepsy nurse, GP)
- Educate the patient and family about the condition

Sodium valproate side effects

VALPROAT²E: **V**ery potent enzyme inhibitor, **A**ppetite ↑, **L**iver failure, **P**ancreatitis, **R**eversible hair loss, **O**edema, **A**taxia, **T**eratogenicity/**T**remor, **E**ncephalopathy (↑ ammonia)

Carbamazepine side effects

HARD SAND: **H**eadache, **A**taxia, **R**ash, **D**izziness, **S**exual dysfunction, **A**naemia, **N**ausea, **D**iplopia

Carbamazepine is an enzyme **inducer**, valproate is an enzyme **inhibitor**.

- For women, counsel about pregnancy (as they may be taking teratogenic medications; see box):
  - There are specific guidelines around the use of valproate in women of childbearing age → a pregnancy prevention programme must be in place
- Inform the patient that they must contact the DVLA
- Assess the person's risk of osteoporosis if they are taking antiepileptic drugs
- Annual risk assessment including factors that may lessen their risk of sudden unexpected death in epilepsy (SUDEP)

Pharmacological

- The type of antiepileptic varies depending on the type of seizures the patient has, their age and comorbidities. In general:
  - If generalised seizures → first line: **sodium valproate** (**unless female**); second line: lamotrigine (may aggravate myoclonus), levetiracetam
  - If focal seizures → first line: **levetiracetam** or lamotrigine; second line: carbamazepine

Surgical

- If a structural epileptogenic focus can be identified (such as hippocampal sclerosis or tumour), then neurosurgical resection can be potentially curative. Vagus nerve stimulation is also used.

REFERENCE

National Institute for Health and Care Excellence. NICE Guidelines, Epilepsy. https://cks.nice.org.uk/epilepsy)

6.4 MULTIPLE SCLEROSIS

DEFINITION

Multiple sclerosis (MS) is a chronic, autoimmune inflammatory condition of the central nervous system (CNS) characterised by demyelination of the white matter.

EPIDEMIOLOGY

MS typically arises in young adults (20–40 years). It is three times more common in women and more common at extremes of latitude.

AETIOLOGY

The aetiology of MS remains unclear but there are a number of risk factors, such as Epstein–Barr virus infection, smoking, female gender and geographical location. There is a genetic component to MS, with an increased relative risk in offspring of affected parents compared to the general population.

PATHOLOGY

Inflammation results in areas of demyelination affecting the white matter anywhere in the CNS, leading to neuronal damage.

CLINICAL PRESENTATION

Symptoms vary according to the area affected, but typical sites affected are optic nerve (causing optic neuritis), brainstem (varied signs but typically diplopia with an intranuclear ophthalmoplegia, vertigo and nystagmus) with or without cerebellar involvement, spinal cord (causing a transverse myelitis resulting in a spastic paraparesis, sensory loss, urinary incontinence) or cerebral hemispheres (varied symptoms, e.g. hemisensory loss or hemiparesis).

There are three main patterns of MS:

- Relapsing–remitting MS (85% of patients): Episodes of symptoms are followed by recovery and periods of stability. There may be residual damage to parts of the CNS that results in only a partial recovery during remissions
- Secondary progressive MS: Occurs typically 15–20 years after onset of relapsing–remitting MS with gradual worsening of neurological function, with or without continued relapses
- Primary progressive MS (10%–15% of patients): There is a steady gradual worsening of the disease from the onset, without remissions

To diagnose MS, there needs to be evidence of dissemination of lesions of the CNS in both time and space. The revised **MacDonald criteria** is used to diagnose MS. The MacDonald criteria aims to establish that lesions have developed at different times in different anatomical locations.

EXAMINATION

As MS affects the upper motor neurons (UMN) you should look for these signs in examination:

- Increased muscle tone
- Weakness (generally flexors stronger than extensors in the arms and reverse in the legs – this is known as a pyramidal pattern of weakness)
- Brisk reflexes
- Up-going plantar response

Examine the eyes, cranial nerves, sensation and cerebellar function to check for a cerebellar syndrome (see 6.7).

> **Tip**: In a UMN lesion everything goes up (muscle tone, plantars, reflexes).

INVESTIGATIONS

Bloods: Aquaporin 4 antibodies (causes NMO – neuromyelitis optica, a MS mimicker), vitamin B_{12} (deficiency can cause dorsal column abnormalities and peripheral neuropathy), HIV screen (can cause encephalopathy and myelopathy), ESR (screen for inflammatory conditions, such as SLE and sarcoidosis).

Imaging: MRI head and spinal cord to detect areas of demyelination and to exclude cord compression.

Invasive: CSF may show unmatched oligoclonal IgG bands.

DIFFERENTIAL DIAGNOSIS

The most common differential diagnosis for MS with limb symptoms is compressive myelopathy – therefore it is essential to request an MRI to rule out cervical cord compression.

The differential diagnosis for MS includes other demyelinating disease (NMO), metabolic disorders (vitamin B_{12} and copper deficiency), infections (HIV, tertiary syphilis), inflammatory disorders (SLE, Behçet's syndrome, sarcoidosis) or neoplasia (primary/metastatic/paraneoplastic).

MANAGEMENT

Non-pharmacological

- Multidisciplinary team care (MS specialist nurse, neurologist, occupational therapist, physiotherapist and GP involvement)
- Education about the condition and signposting to organisation such as the MS Trust and Society

Pharmacological

- Relapse management: Methylprednisolone (oral or IV) for 5 days
- Disease-modifying drugs: Aim to reduce relapses rates and/or induce remission:
  - Monoclonal antibodies (alemtuzumab, ocrelizumab)
  - Oral drugs (cladribine, fingolimod, teriflunomide, dimethylfumarate), intravenous (natalizumab)

- Subcutaneous (beta-interferon, glatiramer acetate)
- Management of complications:
  - Fatigue:
    - Exclude other causes (anaemia, depression, hypothyroidism etc.)
    - Offer information regarding overexertion and regular exercise
    - Consider interventions such as CBT and mindfulness
    - Consider a trial of amantadine
  - Spasticity:
    - Assess for triggers for spasms (such as constipation, urinary tract infections, pain)
    - Consider anti-spasticity drugs such as baclofen
  - Mobility:
    - Asses for factors that may reduce mobility (fatigue, spasticity and visual problems)
    - Refer for assessment for a supervised exercise programme or mobility aid
  - Depression:
    - Consider offering non-pharmacological interventions such as CBT
    - Pharmacological interventions such as SSRIs
- Pain:
  - Musculoskeletal pain may benefit from physiotherapy or simple NSAID analgesia
  - Neuropathic pain may require agents such as gabapentin, amitriptyline, pregabalin or duloxetine
- Memory impairment:
  - Usually multi-factorial from a direct effect of MS, depression, side effects of medications and fatigue. Compensatory strategies, e.g. list making, setting a routine may help. More formal cognitive rehabilitation can be used in more severe cases
- Bladder and bowel problems (incontinence):
  - Conservative measures can be considered such as lifestyle advice, fluid intake and the use of absorbent products/pads. Incontinence teams can be involved for pharmacological and more invasive management
- Sexual function:
  - Patients should be considered for the option of relationship or psychosexual counselling if appropriate. Men may be eligible to have medication for erectile dysfunction

6.5 MIGRAINE/HEADACHE

DEFINITION

Migraine is a common primary headache disorder characterised by moderate-severe recurrent headaches with associated symptoms such as nausea, photophobia and phonophobia. There are different types of migraine – these can be broadly divided into migraine with aura and migraine without aura.

EPIDEMIOLOGY

Migraines are three times more common in women.

AETIOLOGY/PATHOLOGY

The exact cause and pathological process of migraines are not well understood. There is a significant genetic component to migraine (a first-degree relative has migraines in 50% of cases).

CLINICAL PRESENTATION

Patients typically give an account of recurrent, moderate-severe headaches that last for hours, up to 3 days. This headache may be unilateral and pulsating in nature and may be associated with gastrointestinal symptoms such as nausea and vomiting. There may be associated photophobia or phonophobia. The headaches limit their activities and patients often retreat to a dark and quiet environment until the headache subsides.

About one-third of patients with migraines have an associated aura. Typically, this is a visual aura that occurs 5–60 minutes before the headache, where a patient has a transient hemianopic disturbance or a spreading scintillating scotoma. Other focal neurological disturbances may be present, such as dysphasia or unilateral paraesthesia. The key factor to obtain in the history is that the neurological disturbance is transient and spreading. It is well recognised that a migrainous aura can occur sometimes without subsequent headache, a situation that can cause confusion with other conditions, e.g. TIA.

EXAMINATION

Many primary causes of headache are diagnosed from specific features in the history (Table 6.5.1).

For any patient with a headache, a physical examination should include ophthalmoscopy (to rule out papilloedema), examination of the head and neck (to rule out cervicogenic headache) and BP measurement.

Importantly, you should look out for the features of the serious secondary causes of a headache (meningitis, giant cell arteritis, raised intracranial pressure, SAH).

INVESTIGATIONS

Investigations are of little help for diagnosing primary headaches but can be useful when a secondary headache is suspected (e.g. ESR for temporal arteritis, CT head if SAH or SOL is suspected).

DIFFERENTIAL DIAGNOSIS

The differential diagnosis for a headache is wide (Table 6.5.1). The most common differentials include tension-type headache and cluster headache. The diagnostic criteria are different depending on the presence/absence of aura.

Migraine **with** aura: Two or more attacks with:

- One or more symptoms of aura including visual/sensory symptoms or dysphasia
- Aura lasts <60 minutes

Migraine **without** aura: Five attacks with the following:

- Headaches that last 4–72 hours
- Two of the following: Unilateral location, moderate/severe pain, pulsating quality, aggravation by routine physical activity
- At least one of: Nausea/vomiting or photophobia/phonophobia
- Headache not attributed to a secondary headache disorder

MANAGEMENT

Non-pharmacological

- Use a headache diary to identify potential triggers for migraines (e.g. stress, foods, dehydration)
- Counsel about the risk of medication-overuse headache (MOH) with frequent use of analgesics
- Acupuncture can be considered if preventative medications are ineffective or unsuitable

Pharmacological

- **Acute treatment**: Combination therapy with an oral triptan and simple analgesia (paracetamol/ibuprofen)
- Antiemetic can be prescribed (even in the absence of nausea or vomiting)
- **Preventative treatment**: Consider if >2 attacks per month or cause disability lasting >3 days or if triptans or analgesia are contraindicated or ineffective:
  - Propranolol: Suitable if the patient has coexisting hypertension or anxiety, CI in asthma
  - Topiramate: Avoid prescribing in women of childbearing age as teratogenic and is an enzyme inducer so ↓ effectiveness of hormonal contraceptives
  - Acupuncture and riboflavin may be effective as preventative treatments
  - Botulinum toxin injections: If patient has tried three preventatives with no benefit and is not overusing analgesics

Table 6.5.1 Differential diagnosis of acute headache

Headache	History	Examination	Investigations	Management
Tension-type headache (primary)	Bilateral tight-band sensation Associated with stress Recurrent	Tension and tenderness in neck	None required	Simple analgesics Avoid triggers
Cluster headache (primary)	Painful attacks around one eye Pain is very severe Patient is very restless with the pain (in contrast with migraine) Attacks last <3 hours May occur daily for up to 3 months Associated lacrimation/flushing	Lacrimation Swollen eyelid	None required	Oxygen Triptans for acute Preventative verapamil
Medication-overuse headache (primary)	Regular intake of analgesics (even paracetamol + aspirin) Worse in morning/awakening	Often normal	None required	Stop analgesics for headache!
Trigeminal neuralgia (secondary)	Stabbing pain in trigeminal nerve distribution Triggers (e.g. shaving)	Normal	MRI head to look for MS (in young) and neurovascular compression of the trigeminal nerve	Carbamazepine
Meningitis (secondary) (see Section 9.2)	Systemically unwell (rash, fever) Photophobia Neck stiffness	Photophobia Kernig's and Brudzinski's positive Non-blanching rash	Blood culture Lumbar puncture	IV antibiotics (3rd generation cephalosporins) IM benzylpenicillin if in community Corticosteroids
Temporal arteritis (secondary)	Unilateral scalp throbbing pain Older patient (>55) Scalp tenderness Jaw claudication, vision change	Temporal tenderness, ipsilateral blindness	ESR ($\uparrow\uparrow$) Temporal artery biopsy	High-dose corticosteroids
Subarachnoid haemorrhage (secondary)	Sudden severe headache Meningism	Nuchal rigidity	CT head Lumbar puncture >12 h if CT normal	Interventional radiology or neurosurgery
Raised ICP (secondary)	Progressive symptoms Worse on coughing/laughing Visual disturbance Worse in morning/awakening	↓ GCS Papilloedema Cushing response	CT head AVOID LP	Treat cause (e.g. tumour/hydrocephalus)
Acute closed angle glaucoma (secondary)	Pain around one eye Red, swollen eye Visual blurring and halos	↓ Visual acuity Cloudy cornea Pupil mid-dilated and irregular	Tonometry (>24 mmHg)	Pilocarpine drops IV acetazolamide
Sinusitis (secondary)	Facial pain Postural element (worse on leaning forwards) Rhinorrhoea/nasal congestion	Sinus tenderness	None required ENT referral if diagnosis uncertain	Antibiotics Saline nasal drops Simple analgesia
Idiopathic intracranial hypertension (secondary)	Subacute onset Headache worse in the morning Nausea + vomiting Pulsatile tinnitus ↑ Body weight	Papilloedema Cranial nerve abnormalities (VI)	CT/MRI-venogram to exclude mass lesions and venous sinus thrombosis. LP to measure opening pressure (>25 cmCSF)	LP to relieve pressure Weight loss Acetazolamide

6.6 NEUROPATHIES

POLYNEUROPATHIES

Definition

Polyneuropathies are disorders of the peripheral or cranial nerves. They can be classified by time course (acute/chronic), underlying pathology (demyelinating/axonal) or whether they cause a predominantly motor or sensory loss.

Aetiology

Predominantly **motor loss** (demyelinating):

- Gulliain–Barré syndrome (GBS)
- Chronic inflammatory demyelinating polyneuropathy (CIDP)
- Charcot–Marie–Tooth (hereditary sensorimotor neuropathy)

Predominantly **sensory loss** (**ABCDE**) (axonal):

- **A**lcohol
- **B**$_{12}$ deficiency
- **C**hronic kidney disease
- **D**rugs/diabetes
- **E**very vasculitis

Malignancy is also a common cause of polyneuropathy (commonly lung cancer, myeloma and lymphoma).

Drugs causing polyneuropathy include amiodarone, isoniazid, nitrofurantoin, metronidazole and chemotherapy.

Pathology

The common pathological processes are outlined here.

As a general rule, conditions that cause a predominantly motor loss are caused by **demyelination** whereas conditions that cause a predominantly sensory loss are caused by **axonal** degeneration.

GBS: Immune-mediated demyelination of the peripheral nervous system by antibodies, often triggered by infection (*Campylobacter jejuni*). Anti-GM1 antibodies occur in 25% of patients (especially in acute motor forms).

Alcoholic neuropathy: Secondary to toxic effects and ↓ absorption of B vitamins.

Vitamin B$_{12}$ deficiency: Axonal pathology that may lead to subacute combined degeneration of the cord.

Diabetic neuropathy and vasculitis: Damage to the blood vessels to neurons, leading to demyelination.

Clinical Presentation

The presentation will depend on the underlying cause. Generally speaking, polyneuropathies often cause symmetrical, widespread symptoms with the distal areas affected first (e.g. glove and stocking distribution).

Specific questions to ask include timing, whether symptoms are predominantly motor or sensory in nature and whether there were any preceding events (e.g. infection with *Campylobacter* classically occurs prior to GBS, weight loss in malignancy). Motor symptoms include weakness, falls, respiratory difficulty (e.g. in GBS).

GBS classically has an **ascending** weakness. Sensory symptoms include numbness, neuropathic pain, paraesthesia, joint deformity and sensory ataxia.

Examination

A full neurological examination should be performed to assess the degree of motor and sensory loss, which should be mapped out to indicate the distribution. There may be signs on examination indicating the underlying cause (e.g. tremor, AV fistula in CKD). Specific neurological findings on examination may include:

- GBS: Weakness in all four limbs, mild sensory signs, areflexia, cranial nerve involvement (diplopia)
- LMN signs include: Hypotonia, hyporeflexia and less commonly fasciculations

Investigations

Bedside: Urinalysis (vasculitis, renal failure), nerve conduction studies, spirometry (respiratory function).

Bloods: FBC (infection, anaemia), U&Es (CKD), LFTs (alcohol), blood glucose (DM), B$_{12}$ (↓), immunology (ANA/ANCA for vasculitis), bone profile (↑ Ca^{2+} in myeloma), ESR (vasculitis/myeloma), protein electrophoresis.

Imaging: CXR/CT if malignancy suspected.

Invasive: LP (may be performed if CIDP or GBS suspected), lymph node biopsy (lymphoma).

Management

Treat the underlying cause.

Non-pharmacological

Physiotherapy, OT and podiatry can help minimise trauma and aid mobility.

Pharmacological

Steroids for vasculitis may help. Steroids or IV immunoglobulin for GBS and CIDP.

Treatment options for neuropathic pain include amitriptyline, pregabalin, gabapentin and duloxetine.

MONONEUROPATHIES

Definition

Mononeuropathies are lesions of individual peripheral or cranial nerves.

Cranial nerve lesions

Third nerve palsy

- Features: 4 Ds: Eye is **d**eviated **d**own and out, with a **d**ilated pupil and a **d**ropping eyelid (ptosis).

- Causes: DM, vasculitis, microvascular disease, MS, Weber's syndrome (occurs with contralateral hemiplegia by midbrain stroke), amyloidosis, posterior communicating artery aneurysm (often painful and referred to as a 'surgical third nerve palsy').

Sixth nerve palsy

- Features: Failure of **abduction** of the affected eye leading to diplopia.
- Causes: Idiopathic, DM, trauma, ↑ ICP, MS, nasopharyngeal carcinoma, microvascular disease.

Facial nerve palsy

- Features: Weakness of muscles of facial expression leading to a dropped face, altered taste (anterior 2/3 tongue), failure of eye closure, hyperacusis (CN VII supplies nerve to stapedius in the middle ear)
- Causes:
  - Bilateral: Sarcoidosis, GBS, Lyme disease, neurofibromatosis type II (bilateral acoustic neuromas)
  - Unilateral: Ask the patient to raise their forehead and close their eyes to differentiate between UMN and LMN. In UMN, forehead is spared as there is bilateral cortical supply
    - LMN: **Bell's palsy (most common cause)**, acoustic neuroma, DM, MS, parotid tumours, HIV, Ramsay–Hunt syndrome (reactivation of herpes zoster virus)
    - UMN: Stroke
- Investigations: Blood glucose (DM), HIV testing, serology for *Borrelia* (Lyme), ↑ VZV antibodies (Ramsay–Hunt syndrome), MRI (may show tumour/acoustic neuroma)
- Treatment:
  - Treat the underlying cause (if one found)
  - Treatment for Bell's palsy involves giving prednisolone if <72 h of onset followed by eye protection (artificial tears, dark glasses). Most cases recover spontaneously within 9 months

Median nerve hand supply

LOAF:

Lateral two lumbricals

Opponens pollicis

Abductor pollicis brevis

Flexor pollicis brevis

Carpal tunnel syndrome causes:

MEDIAN TRAP:

Myoxedema

o**E**dema

Diabetes

Idiopathic by far the most common

Acromegaly

Neoplasm

Trauma

Rheumatoid arthritis

Amyloidosis

Pregnancy

Peripheral nerve lesions

Median nerve

C6–T1 (most common mononeuropathy)

- Features: Weakness of precision grip and sensory loss of radial 3.5 fingers
- Causes: Tinel's test and Phalen's test may be positive
- Treatment: Splinting, local steroid injections, decompression surgery

Ulnar nerve

C7–T1

- Features: Weakness of the wrist/hand muscles; clawing of ring/little finger
- Causes: Trauma at medial epicondyle, cubital tunnel syndrome, Guyon's canal, the hand (between pisform and hamate)

Lateral cutaneous nerve of the thigh

- L2–L3 (Meralgia paraesthetica)
- Features: Anterolateral burning thigh pain
- Causes: Entrapment under the inguinal ligament

Common peroneal nerve

L4–S1

- Features: **foot drop**: Test by asking the patient to dorsiflex against resistance
- Causes: Trauma to the fibula head

6.7 CEREBELLAR SYNDROME

DEFINITION

A cerebellar syndrome occurs due to dysfunction of the cerebellum. Lesions may affect the cerebellum directly, via **input** to the cerebellum from proprioceptors, vestibular receptors and cerebral hemispheres via the inferior and middle cerebellar peduncles or the **output** from cerebellum via the superior cerebellar peduncles.

AETIOLOGY

There are a number of conditions that can cause a cerebellar syndrome, which can be remembered by the mnemonic **DAISIES**: **D**emyelination, **A**lcohol, **I**nfarct, **S**pace-occupying lesion, **I**nherited (Friedreich's ataxia), **E**pilepsy medication, **S**ystem atrophy (multiple).

CLINICAL PRESENTATION

The presentation of cerebellar syndrome varies depending on the causative condition and the location of the lesion.

Lesions of the midline vermis tend to cause truncal ataxia whereas lesions of an individual hemisphere typically cause ipsilateral limb ataxia.

There may be other localising brainstem signs such as cranial nerve palsies if the cerebellopontine angle is involved (Figure 6.7.1).

EXAMINATION

Observation: General – does the patient have any **resting neurological signs** (e.g. tremor) or do they use a wheelchair?

- Gait: Ask the patient to walk (including heel-toe) – remember to walk with them in case they fall (assessing for **ataxic gait**).
- **Romberg test**: Ask the patient to close their eyes and stand with their feet together (assessing for **sensory ataxia**).

Face:

- Eyes:
  - Perform the 'H' test to test **extraocular muscle function**
  - While testing, pause when your finger is out laterally to look for **nystagmus**
  - Put two fingers out and ask the patient to look from one finger to another to look for **hypometric saccades**
- Speech: Assess for **slurred/staccato speech** by asking the patient to say a phrase such as 'baby hippopotamus' or 'West register street'

Upper limb:

- Assess muscle tone looking for evidence of **hypotonia**
- Perform the **rebound test**: Ask the patient to hold their arms out fully extended with the palms facing upwards and push their wrists down briskly and quickly let go. If there is evidence of the arms accentuating upward then this is **cerebellar drift** (indicating an ipsilateral cerebellar lesion)
- Assess co-ordination:
  - Ask the patient to slap one hand in the other looking for **dysdiadokokinesis**
  - Perform the **finger–nose test** looking for evidence of an intention tremor

Lower limb:

- Assess muscle tone looking for evidence of **hypotonia**
- Assess co-ordination (**heel–shin test**)
- Ideally:
  - Perform **ophthalmoscopy**, looking for **papilloedema** (a sign of a space occupying lesion)
  - Perform a full neurological examination and examine the cranial nerves, especially **CN V, VII and VIII** to exclude a **cerebellopontine angle lesion**

INVESTIGATIONS

Bloods: FBC, LFTs, TFTs, vitamin E, coeliac antibodies, anti-Hu antibodies, genetic testing (e.g. Friedreich's ataxia).

Imaging: MRI head.

MANAGEMENT

Management will depend on the causative condition. See the following for more details:

Diabetes (4.1), Stroke (6.1), Wilson's (3.5), MS (6.4).

> ### Cerebellar signs
>
> **DANIS²H**: **D**ysdiadochokinesis, **A**taxia, **N**ystagmus, **I**ntention tremor, **S**lurred/**S**taccato speech, **H**ypotonia

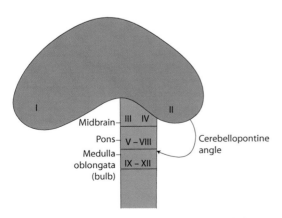

Figure 6.7.1 Location of cranial nerve nuclei and the cerebellopontine angle.

NEUROLOGY: QUESTIONS

6.1 STROKE/TIA

1. Name three risk factors for an ischaemic stroke.
2. Within what time frame of stroke symptoms should thrombolysis be given in an ischaemic stroke, provided there are no contraindications?

6.2 PARKINSON'S DISEASE

1. Name three causes of parkinsonism.
2. Name three features of parkinsonism.

6.3 EPILEPSY

Vanessa is a 27-year-old woman who suffers with generalised tonic–clonic seizures that are managed with sodium valproate.

1. Name two side effects of sodium valproate.
2. Vanessa is interested in driving again. How long does she need to be seizure free before being able to drive?

6.4 MULTIPLE SCLEROSIS

1. What are the different patterns of multiple sclerosis?
2. What are the complications of multiple sclerosis?

6.5 MIGRAINE/HEADACHE

1. What features in a headache history support a diagnosis of migraine?
2. What medication can be offered to patients as prophylaxis for migraine attacks?

6.6 NEUROPATHIES

1. Guillain–Barré syndrome classically has what features on examination?
2. What are the causes of carpal tunnel syndrome?

6.7 CEREBELLAR SYNDROME

1. Name three signs of cerebellar syndrome that can be elicited on examination.
2. Name three causes of cerebellar syndrome.

Renal and Electrolytes

7.1 ACUTE KIDNEY INJURY

DEFINITION

Acute kidney injury (AKI) describes a reduction in renal function following an insult to the kidneys. It is diagnosed by meeting one of three criteria (Table 7.1.1):

- A rise in serum creatinine of 26 μmol/L or greater within 48 hours
- A 50% or greater rise in serum creatinine to have occurred within the past 7 days
- A fall in urine output to less than 0.5 mL/kg/h for more than 6 hours

AETIOLOGY/PATHOLOGY

The causes of AKI can be divided into prerenal, intrinsic renal, and postrenal (Table 7.1.2).

The most common causes of AKI are **prerenal** and **acute tubular necrosis** (**ATN**). These can be differentiated by urine osmolality and urinary sodium. In prerenal AKI, the concentrating powers of the kidney are retained, so **urine osmolality is high and urinary sodium is low** (as it is being reabsorbed). In ATN, the concentrating powers of the kidney are lost, meaning that the **urine osmolality is isotonic to the plasma and that urinary sodium is high** (due to the inability of the kidneys to reabsorb it). The urine in ATN is also described as being 'muddy brown'.

The insult to the kidneys means that it cannot perform its regular functions. The problems from AKI can be summarised as:

- Uraemia
- Failure of fluid balance (fluid overload)

Table 7.1.1 The RIFLE criteria for grading AKI

Stage	Criteria
1	Creatinine rise of 26 μmol or more within 48 hours OR Creatinine rise of 50%–99% from baseline within 7 days OR Urine output <0.5 mL/kg/h for more than 6 hours
2	100%–199% creatinine rise from baseline within 7 days OR Urine output <0.5 mL/kg/h for more than 12 hours
3	200% or more creatinine rise from baseline within **7 days** OR Urine output <0.3 mL/kg/h for 24 hours or anuria for 12 hours OR Any requirement for renal replacement therapy

- Failure of electrolyte regulation (↑ K$^+$)
- Failure of acid–base regulation (metabolic acidosis)

CLINICAL PRESENTATION

Oliguria is a common finding for patients with AKI. Other symptoms depend on the cause of the AKI.

EXAMINATION

Examination should involve a volume status examination as well as identifying the cause of the AKI.

A volume status examination consists of pulse measurement, BP, capillary refill time, JVP measurement, temperature and assessment of mucous membranes and skin turgor. Passive leg raising can also be used – with the patient lying down their legs are raised to 45°. If after 30–90 seconds they show no signs of haemodynamic improvement, it indicates that volume replacement may be required.

INVESTIGATIONS

Bedside: Urinalysis + culture (infection, protein, blood), ECG (looking for ECG evidence of hyperkalaemia – see Section 7.4), fluid balance chart.

Bloods: FBC (infection), U&Es (renal function, K$^+$), blood cultures and lactate (if sepsis suspected), ABG (metabolic acidosis), autoantibody screen (ANA, ANCA, anti-GBM).

Imaging: Ultrasound (exclude obstruction and assess renal size), CXR (pulmonary oedema).

Invasive: Biopsy (if renal cause suspected).

There are many renal causes of an AKI that may come up in clinical scenarios in your written examinations. Table 7.1.3 provides clinical scenarios describing conditions that can cause an AKI.

MANAGEMENT

Treat the complications: Hyperkalaemia, pulmonary oedema, acidosis, dehydration (if present).

Treat the cause if present, e.g. fluid resuscitation if prerenal caused by sepsis.

Table 7.1.2 Causes of AKI

Prerenal	Renal	Postrenal
Hypovolaemia Reduced cardiac output	Nephrotoxic drugs Vascular (vasculitis, thrombosis) Glomerular (glomerulonephritis) Tubular (ischaemic – ATN, rhabdomyolysis, myeloma) Interstitial (interstitial nephritis)	Obstruction (stones, blocked catheter, pelvic mass, enlarged prostate, cervical cancer, retroperitoneal fibrosis)

Table 7.1.3 Examples of conditions causing AKI

Condition	Clinical scenario	Notes
Systemic lupus erythematosus (SLE)	A 41 y/o woman develops oliguria. She has a malar rash and joint pain	SLE can cause proteinuria and glomerulonephritis, most common diffuse proliferative glomerulonephritis
Goodpasture's syndrome	A 26 y/o man presents with shortness of breath, haemoptysis and renal failure. He is found to have an abnormal CXR and a raised total gas transfer factor (TLCO)	Associated with pulmonary haemorrhage and rapidly progressive glomerulonephritis. Caused by antiglomerular basement membrane (anti-GBM) antibodies. Pulmonary haemorrhage can lead to an increased TLCO
Rhabdomyolysis	A 78 y/o woman has a fall and acquires a fractured neck of femur. She was on the floor for 8 hours	Breakdown of muscle by prolonged stay on floor following floor/seizure. Findings include a disproportionately raised creatinine and elevated CK
IgA nephropathy	A 21 y/o man develops haematuria days following a URTI	Most common cause of glomerulonephritis. Differentiated from poststreptococcal glomerulonephritis by the onset following an URTI (days instead of weeks) and complement levels (low in poststreptococcal)
Multiple myeloma	A 68 y/o man presents with a history of severe lower back pain. His latest bloods show ↑ Ca^{2+}	Bence-Jones proteins can be found in the urine
Henoch–Schonlein purpura (HSP)	A 19 y/o man develops oliguria. He has recently developed a lower limb rash, abdominal pain and arthritis	Typically occurs following streptococcal URTI. Triad of abdominal pain, purpuric rash and arthritis
Granulomatosis with polyangitis (GPA)	A 56 y/o woman with a saddle-nose deformity develops epistaxis and haematuria	Vasculitis affecting upper and lower respiratory tract as well as the kidneys. C-ANCA is positive in >90%
Renal cell carcinoma (RCC)	A 77 y/o man is found to have hypertension, haematuria and polycythaemia	Classic triad of haematuria, loin pain and abdominal mass. Metastases via the renal vein to the lung (cannonball metastases). Paraneoplastic effects include polycythaemia (EPO secretion), hypercalcaemia (PTH secretion), hypertension (renin secretion) and Cushing's (ACTH secretion)
Haemolytic uraemic syndrome (HUS)	A 17 y/o girl is found to have an AKI. She has recently had gastroenteritis. Culture grew *E. coli* 0157:H7	Triad of AKI, microangiopathic haemolytic anaemia and thrombocytopenia. Classically caused post-dysentery by *E. coli* 0157:H7. Also, tumours, pregnancy, SLE and HIV

7.2 CHRONIC KIDNEY DISEASE

DEFINITION
Chronic kidney disease (CKD) is an abnormality of kidney function that is present for >3 months. It is diagnosed when tests show a reduction in kidney function or the presence of proteinuria. It is diagnosed when the eGFR drops below 60 mL/min/1.73 m² (see box).

EPIDEMIOLOGY
CKD has an estimated prevalence of 6% in England alone.

AETIOLOGY/PATHOLOGY
The causes of CKD can be remembered by the mnemonic **D²R CABG** (which should also help you remember that patients with CKD are 20 times more likely to die from cardiovascular disease!): **D**iabetes/**D**rugs, **R**enal infection, **C**ongenital (polycystic kidney disease), **A**utoimmune (SLE/vasculitis), **B**lood pressure (hypertension), **G**lomerulonephritis.

CKD is a multisystem disease:

- Nervous system: Peripheral neuropathy, uraemic encephalopathy, fatigue
- Cardiovascular: Accelerated atherogenesis, fluid overload, uraemic pericarditis
- Gastrointestinal: Impaired taste
- Musculoskeletal: Renal osteodystrophy, gout
- Blood: Anaemia (reduced EPO secretion)
- Respiratory: Pulmonary oedema
- Skin: Pruritus (phosphate retention)
- Endocrine: CKD affects sexual hormones and leads to secondary (and potentially tertiary) hyperparathyroidism

The main problems with CKD can be summarised as:

- Failure to **excrete**, leading to uraemia, hyperphosphataemia and hyperkalaemia
- Failure to **regulate**, leading to fluid overload (hypertension and oedema) and metabolic acidosis
- Failure to **create**, leading to anaemia (=EPO) and hypocalcaemia (↓ activated vitamin D)

CLINICAL PRESENTATION
CKD is often an incidental finding on a blood test, but patients may present with fatigue or a complication of the disease.

EXAMINATION
Looking for evidence of the complications of CKD.

Observation: Fluid balance chart, dialysis machine.

Hands: Flapping tremor (uraemia), leukonychia (↓ albumin), fingertip glucose prick marks (diabetes).

Arms: Presence of an arterio-venous fistula (listen for bruit), pulse and blood pressure, yellow skin (uraemia).

Head/neck: Conjunctival pallor (anaemia), arcus lipidus/xanthalasmia (hyperlipidaemia), JVP (fluid overload).

Chest: Heart sounds (uraemic pericarditis), lung sounds (pulmonary oedema).

Abdomen: Scars (Rutherford Morrison in L/RIF if had renal transplant), peritoneal dialysis scar, palpable kidneys (PKD), percussion (ascites), auscultation (renal bruits).

Legs: Peripheral oedema.

INVESTIGATIONS
Bedside: ECG (↑ K⁺, pericarditis), urinalysis (renal failure and to calculate ACR), blood pressure (HTN).

Bloods: FBC (anaemia), U&Es (degree of renal failure, ↑ K⁺), bone profile (↑ PO₄⁻, ↓ Ca²⁺), urate (gout), blood glucose/HbA1c (diabetes), ESR (autoimmune inflammation).

Imaging: Ultrasound scan (kidney size), CT KUB, CXR (pulmonary oedema).

Invasive: Renal biopsy (if glomerulonephritis suspected).

CHRONIC DISEASE MANAGEMENT
Non-pharmacological
- Education about the condition and lifestyle modifications
- Optimise control of comorbidities (i.e. diabetes)
- Low potassium diet
- Low phosphate diet (or phosphate binders)

Staging of chronic kidney disease

Stage	eGFR
1	>90
2	60–89
3a	45–59
3b	30–44
4	15–29
5	<15 or on renal replacement therapy

ACE inhibitors in CKD

ACE inhibitors are usually the first-line medication to treat hypertension in CKD but they are nephrotoxic and can ↓ eGFR.

NICE suggests that a decrease in eGFR up to 25% or a rise in creatinine of up to 30% is acceptable.

Pharmacological

- Antihypertensives:
  - If non-diabetic and ACR <30: In line with normal hypertension guidelines
  - If non-diabetic and ACR >30: ACE inhibitor or ARB
  - If diabetic: ACE inhibitor or ARB
  - Furosemide can be particularly helpful if the eGFR falls <45 and has the benefit of ↓ K⁺
- Cardiovascular risk management:
  - Atorvastatin 20 mg for primary prevention
  - Antiplatelet (e.g. aspirin 75 mg) for secondary prevention
- Erythropoietin analogues (EPO) for anaemia (if suitable)
- Calcium supplementation (e.g. cholecalciferol)
- Consider oral bicarbonate (for metabolic acidosis)
- Renal replacement therapy (haemodialysis/haemofiltration/peritoneal dialysis)

Surgical

- Renal transplant:
  - Requires HLA typing prior to procedure
  - Kidney placed in iliac fossa and anastomosed with iliac vessels
  - Short-term complications include hyperacute rejection (occurs in minutes, due to preexisting antibodies against donor HLA antigens) and acute graft failure (occurs <6 months, usually due to mismatched HLA or opportunistic CMV infection)
  - Chronic graft failure (>6 months, antibodies and cell-mediated mechanisms causing fibrosis)

DIALYSIS

Dialysis describes the use of a semipermeable membrane that acts as a filter with a solution to regulate the fluid and electrolytes in the blood. There are three main forms:

- Haemodialysis: Uses an AV fistula (between radial artery and cephalic vein) with blood flowing from one side of a semipermeable membrane with dialysis solution flowing in the opposite direction. Requires multiple treatments per week. Complications include hypotension, infection, thrombosis (from AV fistula) and dialysis disequilibrium syndrome (cerebral oedema).
- Haemofiltration: Blood flows through a machine through a semipermeable membrane but no dialysis solution is used. Positive hydrostatic pressure pushes fluid across. Complications are similar to haemodialysis but haemofiltration causes less hypotension.
- Peritoneal dialysis: Uses the peritoneum as the semipermeable membrane with access gained via a Tenchkoff catheter through the anterior abdominal wall. Cheaper than haemodialysis/haemofiltration and more flexible for patients. Complications include peritonitis (most commonly due to *Staphylococcus epidermidis*). Contraindications include peritoneal adhesions, abdominal hernias and colostomy.

RENAL OSTEODYSTROPHY AND HYPERPARATHYROIDISM

- Phosphate excretion is insufficient and plasma phosphate rises, **stimulating PTH**
- 1-alpha-hydroxylation of vitamin D is impaired, which reduces calcium absorption and serum calcium, further stimulating PTH
- Rise in PTH (secondary hyperparathyroidism) causes activation of osteoclasts and osteoblasts
- Leads to disorganised bone activity that results in **bone loss/fractures**
- Prolonged secondary hyperparathyroidism may eventually lead to tertiary hyperparathyroidism (due to hyperplasia of the parathyroid glands) that typically occurs in end-stage renal failure

7.3 SODIUM IMBALANCE

HYPONATRAEMIA

Definition

Hyponatraemia is defined as serum sodium concentration of less than 135 mmol/L. Its severity can be graded:

- Mild hyponatraemia: 130–135 mmol/L
- Moderate hyponatraemia: 125–129 mmol/L
- Severe hyponatraemia: <125 mmol/L

Hyponatraemia is the most common electrolyte disorder in clinical practice.

Aetiology/Pathology

There are many causes of hyponatraemia. A helpful way of separating them is by the fluid status of the patient. This also helps to inform the best way of managing the patient. A fluid balance assessment considers a patient's current state of hydration by measuring blood pressure, pulse, skin turgor, JVP and urine output.

- Hypovolaemic hyponatraemia; Patients are clinically dehydrated, and the hyponatraemia is due to the relative depletion of salt to water. Causes include fluid loss (GI losses, burns, sweat, poor intake), renal sodium loss (diuretics), third-space losses (pancreatitis, bowel obstruction) and primary adrenal insufficiency.

- Euvolaemic hyponatraemia: Patients demonstrate no dehydration or oedema. The hyponatraemia is due to an excess of water to salt. Causes include excessive fluid therapy (too much IV fluids), polydipsia, syndrome of inappropriate ADH secretion (SIADH) (see box). Rarely euvolaemic hyponatraemia can be caused by pseudohyponatraemia where ↑ serum lipids cause a ↑ serum volume with a ↓ Na$^+$ and a normal serum osmolality. Therefore, in the presence of a normal plasma osmolality it is recommended to measure serum lipids and protein concentrations.

- Hypervolaemic hyponatraemia: Patients are clinically oedematous. The hyponatraemia is caused by the retention of greater water than salt. Causes include organ failure (cardiac, renal, hepatic).

Clinical presentation

The majority of patients with hyponatraemia are asymptomatic or display non-specific symptoms (fatigue, headache, anorexia). Symptoms are often due to the rate of onset and severity. Rapid changes in sodium/severe hyponatraemia can cause neurological symptoms (↓ GCS, coma, seizures) and cardiac arrest. Chronic hyponatraemia can lead to falls and gait instability.

Examination

A fluid status assessment, in addition to a cardiovascular and respiratory examination, should be included in your assessment to help identify an underlying

---

Causes of SIADH

Malignant causes:

- Lung cancer (small cell)
- Lymphoma

Respiratory causes:

- Pneumonia (especially *Legionella*)
- TB
- Aspergillosis

Neurological causes:

- Meningitis
- Subdural haematoma
- Stroke
- Brain tumour

Drugs:

- Diuretics
- SSRIs
- Antipsychotics
- NSAIDs
- Carbamazepine
- TCAs

---

cause. Check to see if the blood sample was taken from the arm receiving IV fluids, as this can commonly be identified as hyponatraemia.

Investigations

Bedside: BP, urine sodium and osmolality (see box).

Bloods: U&Es (Na$^+$, renal function, ↑ urea if dehydrated), LFTs (hepatic failure), BNP (cardiac failure).

Imaging: CXR (heart failure/lung pathology causing SIADH).

Tests for hyponatraemia

If hypovolaemic hyponatraemia:

- Check urinary Na$^+$: If <20 mmol/L, consider fluid loss as a cause, if >20 mmol/L, consider primary adrenal insufficiency/diuretic use

If euvolaemic hyponatraemia:

- Check urine osmolality and serum osmolality. Not helpful if on diuretics
- If urine osmolality < serum osmolality: Likely to be due to too much IV fluids or polydipsia
- If urine osmolality > serum osmolality: Consider secondary adrenal insufficiency or SIADH

Types of diabetes insipidus

Cranial:
- Idiopathic
- Head injury
- Pituitary surgery

Nephrogenic:
- Genetic
- Drugs (lithium, demeclocycline)

Management

Identify and treat the underlying cause of the hyponatraemia.

Management of the hyponatraemia can also be divided based on the fluid status of the patient:

- Hypovolaemic hyponatraemia: Replace fluids and sodium with 0.9% sodium chloride slowly
- Euvolaemic hyponatraemia: Stop IV fluids/drugs if they are the cause. Otherwise restrict fluid intake. Treatment options include furosemide and demeclocycline (which induces a state of diabetes insipidus to $\uparrow$ Na$^+$)
- Hypervolaemic hyponatraemia: Restrict salt and fluid intake and treat the underlying organ failure

Be cautious when correcting Na$^+$ quickly due to the risk of **central pontine myelinolysis** — an irreversible and potentially fatal pontine demyelination caused by rapid correction of $\downarrow$ Na$^+$. It occurs due to the rapid rise in serum osmolality, leaving brain cells with insufficient time to adjust to the new osmolality, causing a drive of water out of the brain cells.

HYPERNATRAEMIA

Definition

Hypernatraemia is defined as a serum sodium concentration of more than 145 mmol/L.

Aetiology/Pathology

Hypernatraemia usually occurs due to water loss in excess of sodium loss. This can be caused by:

- Reduced fluid intake
- Fluid loss in the absence of water replacement (diarrhoea, vomiting, burns)
- Excessive IV saline replacement
- Diabetes insipidus (a deficiency or insensitivity to ADH, cranial or nephrogenic, see box)
- Osmotic diuresis (e.g. hyperosmotic non-ketotic diabetic coma)
- Primary hyperaldosteronism (suspect if hypertension with hypokalaemia)

Clinical presentation

Patients with hypernatraemia can have symptoms of thirst, lethargy, irritability initially, which may progress to confusion, coma and seizures.

Examination

Patients may have signs of dehydration:
- Dry mucous membranes
- Cool peripheries
- $\downarrow$ Skin turgor
- $\downarrow$ Capillary refill time
- $\downarrow$ Urine output
- Hypotension (may have a postural drop)
- Tachycardia

Investigations

Bedside: BP, urine osmolality.

Bloods: U&Es, blood glucose (osmotic diuresis), plasma osmolality (high plasma osmolality + low urine osmolality is suggestive of diabetes insipidus).

Management

Give water orally or IV 5% dextrose slowly guided by urine output and serum Na$^+$. Take care when reducing Na$^+$ levels, as too fast a reduction can cause cerebral oedema. A general rule is to correct at a rate <0.5 mmol/h.

7.4 POTASSIUM IMBALANCE

HYPERKALAEMIA
Definition
Hyperkalaemia is a raised serum potassium level, which requires urgent treatment when >6.5 mmol/L.

Aetiology/Pathology
The causes of hyperkalaemia can be divided into either those causing (1) reduced renal excretion of K^+ or (2) reduced K^+ uptake into cells (*Table 7.4.1*).

Clinical presentation
Patients frequently do not experience symptoms until K^+ is >7 mmol/L. Symptoms may include chest pain, palpitations, light-headedness and muscle weakness. The patient may go into cardiac arrest without warning if K^+ is very high.

Examination
Often no signs on examination. Potential signs include a fast, irregular tachycardia and muscle weakness.

Investigations
Bedside: DO AN ECG! (see box)

Bloods: U&Es, CK (rhabdomyolysis), urate (if tumour lysis syndrome suspected), digoxin levels, ABG.

Management
Individual Hospital Trust guidelines will vary by region, but generally, if K^+ >6.5 mmol/L or ECG changes are present then treat acutely with:

- IV 10 mL of 10% calcium gluconate (stabilises myocardium)
- IV short-acting insulin and glucose (the insulin drives the potassium intracellularly)
- Nebulised salbutamol (salbutamol also drives potassium intracellularly)
- Stop medications that cause ↑ K^+, e.g spironolactone/ramipril

Hyperkalaemia refractory to medical treatment is an indication for dialysis.

Calcium resonium binds K^+ in the gut and can bring down levels over a few days but is not an urgent treatment.

HYPOKALAEMIA
Definition
Hypokalaemia is a reduced serum potassium level, which rarely occurs in the absence of other pathology.

> ### ECG changes with ↑ K^+
> Small/absent p waves
> Broad and wide QRS
> Tall tented T waves

Aetiology/Pathology
Causes of hypokalaemia include vomiting and diarrhoea, diuretic use, Cushing's syndrome, Conn's syndrome.

Genetic causes of hypokalaemia include Bartter syndrome (autosomal recessive inheritance), Gitelman syndrome (autosomal dominant [AD]), Liddle syndrome (AD) and hypokalaemia periodic paralysis (AD).

Clinical presentation
Palpitations, muscle weakness, hypotonia, hyporeflexia, cramps, light-headedness (arrhythmias).

Investigations
The main investigations needed are an ECG (see box) and U&Es.

Management
Stop the offending drugs. If mild hypokalaemia (>2.5 mmol/L and asymptomatic) give oral K^+ supplementation. If severe (<2.5 mmol/L or symptoms) then give K^+ IV cautiously (no more than 20 mmol/h).

> ### ECG changes with ↓ K^+
> Prolonged PR interval
> Flattened T waves
> U wave (after T wave)
> ST depression
> Peaked P wave

Table 7.4.1 Causes of hyperkalaemia

Reduced renal excretion of K^+	Reduced K^+ uptake into cells
Acute kidney injury (AKI)	Metabolic acidosis
Drugs (ACE inhibitors, ARBs, K^+-sparing diuretics, NSAIDs, trimethoprim)	Digoxin
Primary hypoadrenalism	
Hyperkalaemic distal rental tubular acidosis	

Other causes of hyperkalaemia include:
Rhabdomyolysis, tumour lysis syndrome, burns, artefact (pseudohyperkalaemia)

7.5 CALCIUM IMBALANCE

HYPERCALCAEMIA

Definition

Hypercalcaemia is defined as serum calcium of 2.65 mmol/L or higher on two occasions following correction for serum albumin concentration. It can be classified by severity:

- Mild: 2.65–3.00 mmol/L
- Moderate: 3.01–3.40 mmol/L
- Severe: >3.40 mmol/L

Aetiology/Pathology

There are many causes of hypercalcaemia. Ninety percent of causes are due to either:

- Primary hyperparathyroidism (*Table 7.5.1*)
- Malignancy (most commonly breast cancer, lung cancer and multiple myeloma)

Other causes include sarcoidosis, vitamin D toxicity, thyrotoxicosis, lithium, tertiary hyperparathyroidism, milk-alkali syndrome (ingesting too much calcium product) and familial benign hypocalcinuric hypercalcaemia.

Clinical presentation

The symptoms of hypercalcaemia can be remembered by: '**Bones, stones, groans, thrones and psychic moans**': Bones (bone pain), stones (renal calculi), groans (abdominal pain, tiredness/weakness), thrones (polydipsia, constipation), psychic moans (confusion).

Examination

There may be no findings on clinical examination unless there are signs of the underlying cause, e.g.:

- Breast lump (malignancy)
- Cachexia (malignancy)
- Erythema nodosum (sarcoidosis)
- Signs of thyrotoxicosis (see Section 4.3)

Investigations

Bedside: BP ($\uparrow$), ECG (shortened QT interval), urinary Bence–Jones protein (myeloma), 24-hour urinary Ca^{2+} excretion (for familial hypocalciuric hypercalcaemia).

Bloods: Bone profile ($\uparrow$ Ca^{2+}), parathyroid hormone ($\uparrow$ in primary hyperparathyroidism), U&Es (check renal function and electrolytes à polydipsia), vitamin D ($\uparrow$ in toxicity), blood glucose (polydipsia), FBC (anaemia).

Imaging: CXR (lung cancer), isotope bone scan.

Management

Manage acute symptoms (if >3.5 mmol/L and symptomatic):

- Correct dehydration if present with IV 0.9% saline
- Bisphosphonates can be used to lower Ca^{2+} level

Treat underlying cause.

HYPOCALCAEMIA

Definition

Hypocalcaemia is defined as a serum calcium level <2.3 mmol/L. It occurs far less frequently than hypercalcaemia.

Aetiology/Pathology

The causes of hypocalcaemia can be defined by the phosphate level (*Table 7.5.2*).

Clinical presentation

The symptoms of hypocalcaemia can be remembered by the mnemonic **SPASMODIC**[2]: **S**pasms (muscle twitching, tetany), **P**erioral paraesthaesia, **A**nxiety, **S**eizures, **M**uscle tone ($\uparrow$), **O**rientation impaired and confusion, **D**ermatitis, **I**mpetigo herpetiformis (pustules in pregnancy – rare), **C**ataracts/**C**ardiomyopathy.

Examination

Signs are dependent on severity but can range from paraesthesia to seizures.

Look for evidence of previous thyroid surgery (hypoparathyroidism is a complication).

The two eponymous signs to remember for hypocalcaemia are Chvostek's sign and Trousseau's sign:

- Chvostek's sign: The corner of the mouth twitches with tapping of the facial nerve over the parotid

Table 7.5.1 Differentiating between the types of hyperparathyroidism

	Primary hyperparathyroidism	Secondary hyperparathyroidism	Tertiary hyperparathyroidism
Calcium	$\uparrow$	$\downarrow$	$\uparrow$
PTH	$\uparrow$	$\uparrow$	$\uparrow\uparrow$
Phosphate	$\downarrow$	$\uparrow$	$\uparrow$
Causes	Adenoma (85%) Familial hypocalcinuric hypercalcaemia	Chronic kidney disease	Occurs after long period of secondary hyperparathyroidism (CKD) due to hyperplasia of parathyroid gland

Table 7.5.2 Causes of phosphate imbalance

↑ Phosphate	↔ or ↓ Phosphate
Chronic kidney disease	Osteomalacia
Hypoparathyroidism	Vitamin D deficiency
Pseudohypoparathyroidism	Acute pancreatitis
Acute rhabdomyolysis	Overhydration
Hypomagnesaemia	Respiratory alkalosis

- Trousseau's sign: Wrist and finger flexion on inflating the blood pressure cuff

Investigations

Bedside: ECG (widened QT interval), ophthalmology (cataracts).

Bloods: Bone profile (↓ Ca^{2+} phosphate), parathyroid hormone (↓ in primary hypoparathyroidism, *Table 7.5.3*), vitamin D (↓ in deficiency), blood glucose (paraesthesia), CK (rhabdomyolysis), magnesium (↓), ABG (respiratory alkalosis).

Imaging: USS neck, AXR (acute pancreatitis).

Management

Dependent on symptoms severity. For mild symptoms give oral calcium with daily plasma bone profile. For severe symptoms give 10 mL of 10% calcium gluconate IV over 30 minutes.

Treat underlying causes (e.g. respiratory alkalosis/vitamin D deficiency).

Table 7.5.3 Differentiating between the types of hypoparathyroidism

	Primary hypoparathyroidism	Pseudo-hypoparathyroidism	Pseudopseudo-hypoparathyroidism
Calcium	↓	↓	Normal
PTH	↓	↑	Normal
Phosphate	↑	↓	Normal
Notes	Causes: Post-surgery (thyroid) Autoimmune Infiltration (Wilson's) Genetic causes (DiGeorge syndrome)	Rare – either genetic or due to PTH insensitivity Has characteristic features: • Short stature • Short 4th + 5th metacarpals	Very rare No endocrine abnormality Same morphological features as pseudohypoparathyroidism

RENAL AND ELECTROLYTES: QUESTIONS

7.1 ACUTE KIDNEY INJURY

1. Name three causes of acute kidney injury.
2. Name two signs of acute renal failure you may see on examination.
3. Name the three changes you may see in the U&Es for a patient in an acute kidney injury.

7.2 CHRONIC KIDNEY INJURY

1. Name three causes of chronic kidney disease.
2. An eGFR of 25 corresponds to which stage of chronic kidney disease?
3. Name three medical treatments used in the management of chronic kidney disease.

7.3–7.5 ELECTROLYTE IMBALANCES

1. Name three drugs are associated with hyponatraemia.
2. What are the ECG changes associated with hyperkalaemia?
3. What are the symptoms of hypercalcaemia?

Haematology

8.1 ANAEMIA

DEFINITION

Anaemia is lack of sufficient red blood cells and there-fore haemoglobin (Hb). Biochemically, it is defined as a Hb <13 g/dL in men, <12 g/dL in women. If pregnant, these values change to <11 g/dL (1st trimester) and <10.5 g/dL (2nd/3rd trimester).

CLINICAL PRESENTATION

Patients may be asymptomatic for long periods before developing symptoms. Lethargy, palpitations, exertional dyspnoea, angina and night cramps may occur. Severe anaemia can cause high-output cardiac failure.

Patients may also have symptoms of the underlying cause of their anaemia.

EXAMINATION

General signs of anaemia include pallor, tachycardia, tachypnoea and cardiac bruits.

Cause-specific signs of anaemia include:

- Angular stomatitis, koilonychia with iron deficiency anaemia
- Glossitis, peripheral neuropathy, subacute combined degeneration of the cord with B_{12} deficiency
- Weight gain, bradycardia, slow relaxation of biceps jerk, goitre with hypothyroidism

INVESTIGATIONS

Anyone who is found to have a low Hb on their FBC should have their MCV and haematinics checked.

MANAGEMENT

Treat the cause of anaemia (*Table 8.1.1*). If no cause found, then refer to haematology for specialist investigation.

Specific anaemias
Iron deficiency anaemia (IDA)

Determine the cause of the anaemia, e.g. gastrointestinal loss, gynaecological causes, drugs (NSAIDs), diet.

Blood loss from the GI tract is the most common cause of IDA in adult men and postmenopausal women.

Menorrhagia is the most common cause of IDA in premenopausal women.

Referral guidelines:

- People of any age with dyspepsia who present with IDA (2-week wait referral)
- Men of any age with unexplained IDA and Hb <11 g/dL (2-week wait for GI investigations)
- Non-menstruating women with unexplained IDA with Hb <10 g/dL (2-week wait for GI investigations)
- Unexplained IDA will require GI investigations and the clinical picture should determine urgency

Management:

- Dietary advice and oral iron tablet with FBC checked 2–4 weeks after the start of treatment
- Once levels normalised, treatment continued for 3 months and then stopped with FBC monitoring

Table 8.1.1 Causes of anaemia

	Microcytic	Normocytic	Macrocytic
Causes	Iron deficiency anaemia Thalassaemia	Anaemia of chronic disease Acute haemorrhage Combined iron + folate deficiency Haemolytic anaemia	Vitamin B_{12} deficiency Folate deficiency Haemolytic anaemia Hypothyroidism Liver disease Myelodysplasia Drugs Aplastic/hypoplastic anaemia Multiple myeloma
Further investigations	Ferritin Blood film Iron studies Reticulocyte count Abdominal examination (to check for abdominal /rectal mass) Haemoglobin electrophoresis	Blood film Reticulocyte count Ferritin + B_{12}/folate Direct antiglobulin test (DAT) (for AIHA) CRP/ESR (for inflammation) Renal function (check urea for bleed)	Vitamin B_{12}/folate Blood film Direct antiglobulin test (DAT) Liver function tests Thyroid function tests Immunoglobulins Electrophoresis Serum free light chains Reticulocyte count

Table 8.1.2 Types of inherited haemolytic anaemia

Anaemia	Hereditary spherocytosis	G6PD	Sickle cell anaemia	Thalassaemia
Inheritance	Autosomal dominant	X-linked recessive	Autosomal recessive	Autosomal recessive (major and minor)
Diagnostic test	Osmotic fragility test Hb electrophoresis	G6PD enzyme assay	Sickling test (for HbS) NHS screening	NHS screening programme
History	Neonatal jaundice Gallstones	Neonatal jaundice Gallstones Drugs precipitate haemolysis	Crisis: Bone pain, pleuritic chest pain, splenic infarcts	Depending on genes affected Beta-thalassaemia
Blood film	Spherocytes	Heinz bodies	Sickle cells	Microcytosis
Management	Folate replacement Splenectomy	Avoid triggers (fava beans, drugs)	Supportive Hydroxyurea	B-thalassaemia major: Blood transfusions and iron chelator agents

Vitamin B₁₂ or folate deficiency

Determine the cause of the deficiency (common causes include dietary intake, malabsorption, drugs, pregnancy [folate]).

If a vitamin B_{12} deficiency: Check anti-intrinsic factor antibodies for pernicious anaemia.

If folate deficiency and features of malabsorption: Check tissue transglutaminase for coeliac disease.

Seek haematology help if patients have neurological involvement.

Management:

- Vitamin B_{12} deficiency:
  - Initially administer hydroxocobalamin 1 mg IM on alternative days for 2 weeks followed by 1 mg IM every 3 months
  - If thought to be diet related oral cyanocobalamin tablets can be taken between meals
- Folate deficiency:
  - Dietary advice: Encourage intake of broccoli, asparagus, peas, brown rice
  - Check vitamin B_{12} levels in patients with folate deficiency as treatment can mask underlying B_{12} deficiency and allow neurological disease to develop

---

Drugs causing ↓ vitamin B₁₂

- Colchicine
- Metformin
- Anticonvulsants

Drugs causing ↓ folate

- Anticonvulsants
- Methotrexate
- Sulfasalazine

- Prescribe folic acid 5 mg daily
- Measure FBC after 10 days to confirm response (↑ Hb and ↑ reticulocytes) and then after 8 weeks to confirm normal blood count

Haemolytic anaemias

Suggested by a normocytic/macrocytic anaemia, a raised bilirubin, jaundice and raised LDH.

Blood film may show spherocytes (RBCs with a loss in the membrane due to haemolysis) if immune-mediated haemolytic anaemia or hereditary spherocytosis.

Can be divided into autoimmune haemolytic anaemia (AIHA) and inherited haemolytic anaemias (*Table 8.1.2*).

To check:

- Perform a direct antiglobulin test (DAT) and reticulocyte count
- If ↑ reticulocytes and positive DAT = AIHA

AIHA:

- AIHA can be divided into warm and cold AIHA
  - Warm AIHA is mediated by IgG. Causes: Autoimmune conditions (e.g. SLE), lymphoproliferative disorders, drugs
  - Cold AIHA is mediated by IgM. Causes: Infections (EBV, mycoplasma), lymphoma
- Treatment involves corticosteroids, immunosuppression, immunoglobulins, rituximab and rarely splenectomy (for warm AIHA)

Inherited haemolytic anaemia

- The main inherited haemolytic anaemias can be categorised by the affected part of the RBC:
  - Cell membrane: Hereditary spherocytosis/elliptocystosis
  - Cell cytoplasm: Glucose-6-phosphate deficiency (G6PD)
  - Haemoglobin: Sickle cell anaemia, thalassaemia

8.2 HAEMATOLOGICAL MALIGNANCIES

Haematological malignancies include leukaemias, lymphoma, myeloproliferative disorders and multiple myeloma. There is NICE Guidance available for when you may suspect a haematological malignancy.

Arrange urgent FBC and specialist assessment in any adult/child with unexplained fever, persistent infection, generalised lymphadenopathy, unexplained bruising or bleeding and hepatosplenomegaly.

When considering referral, take into account any associated symptoms, particularly fever, night sweats, shortness of breath, pruritus or weight loss.

LEUKAEMIAS

Group of malignant disorders from a single cell affecting all age groups. Leukaemias are divided into lymphocyte (acute lymphoblastic, chronic lymphocytic) or myeloid (acute and chronic myeloid).

Acute leukaemia (ALL and AML)
- Abnormal proliferation of progenitor cells
- Clinical presentation: Symptoms/signs arise from bone marrow failure (anaemia, neutropenia, thrombocytopenia,) and organ infiltration (lymphadenopathy, hepatosplenomegaly)
- Investigations: FBC (↑WCC [due to increased blasts] with ↓ neutrophils), blood film (abnormal with blast cells), CXR (may show mediastinal mass)
- Differentiating factors between ALL and AML:
  - ALL typically occurs in children (ALL is the most common cancer in childhood)
  - AML typically occurs in adulthood and classically has Auer rods present on blood film
- Management:
  - Urgent referral for diagnosis and haematology input
  - Chemotherapy and radiotherapy ± bone marrow transplant

Chronic leukaemia (CLL and CML)
- Abnormal proliferation of lymphocytes/myeloid cells
- Clinical presentation:
  - CLL occurs in the elderly who have widespread painless lymphadenopathy, ↑ lymphocytes on FBC
  - CML occurs at 30–60 years in patients who have non-specific symptoms (↓ weight, anaemia) with splenomegaly, ↑ WCC on FBC
  - Investigations: Testing for the Philadelphia chromosome (9,22 translocation) can help differentiate between the two – Philadelphia chromosome is present in CML

- Management:
  - CLL has good prognosis so once diagnosis is confirmed patients have regular FBC with review and have infections treated promptly. Specialist treatment includes chemotherapy/radiotherapy
  - CML has a good prognosis with tyrosine kinase inhibitors. Upon suspicion of CML, an urgent referral to haematology is required. Treatment is determined by the phase of the disease and involves tyrosine kinase inhibitors (**imatinib**)

LYMPHOMAS
Lymphomas are cancers of the lymphatic system and are divided into Hodgkin's and non-Hodgkin's lymphoma (NHL).

NHL
- Derived from malignant transformation of lymphocytes (85% B cells)
- Fifth most common cancer in the UK. Majority of patients are >60 years old
- Many types. Broadly divided into high-grade and low-grade NHLs. Diffuse large B cell is the most common high-grade NHL, while follicular is the most common low-grade NHL
- Clinical presentation: Painless lymphadenopathy, splenomegaly, ↓ weight, night sweats, fever
- Investigations: FBC, monospot, ESR, LFTs, CXR (mediastinal mass), lymph node biopsy
- Management: Chemotherapy, radiotherapy and, if B cell, rituximab (CD20, anti-B cell)

Hodgkin's lymphoma
- Much rarer than NHL. Peak age range 15–35 and 50–70 years. Derived from B lymphocytes
- **Reed-Sternberg cells** are classically found in affected lymph nodes
- Clinical presentation: Painless lymphadenopathy, splenomegaly (30%), ↓ weight, night sweats, fever
- Investigations and management: As for NHL. Targeted antibody is brentuximab (CD30), which is usually only used after several lines of chemotherapy

MYELOPROLIFERATIVE DISORDERS
Proliferation of >1 of the haemopoietic components of the bone marrow.

POLYCYTHAEMIA RUBRA VERA (↑ HB)
- Features: Night sweats, itching (after a bath), splenomegaly, hypertension. **JAK2 mutation +**
- Increased risk of thromboembolic events. If symptomatic, regular venesection occurs to reduce the number of circulating red blood cells

- Management: Low-dose aspirin (preventing thrombosis) and chemotherapy agents such as interferon alpha (slows down the rate at which blood cells are made) and hydroxycarbamide can also be used. Stem cell/bone marrow transplant can be used for certain individuals

ESSENTIAL THROMBOCYTOSIS (↑ PLATELETS)

- ↑ Risk of thrombosis but very occasionally may have haemorrhage due to ↓ platelet function
- ↑ Risk of thromboembolic events, treated with aspirin
- High-risk patients treated with hydroxycarbamide

MYELOFIBROSIS

- Accumulation of fibrosis tissue in bone marrow. Occurs due to a clonal abnormality of megakaryocytes that produce proinflammatory cytokines (such as fibroblast growth factor), which leads to the replacement of haemopoietic bone marrow tissue by connective tissue. A decrease in haemopoietic tissue leads to progressive bone marrow failure. These changes can lead to a leucoerythroblastic blood film
- Extramedullary haemopoiesis can occur where blood cells are formed outside the bone marrow in areas such as the liver and spleen, leading to hepatomegaly and splenomegaly
- Causes pancytopenia, recurrent infections, fever ± gout. Can transform to AML
- Treatment for symptomatic patients: Blood transfusions and chemotherapy with medications such as hydroxycarbamide, thalidomide or JAK inhibitors. Interferon alpha, EPO, splenectomy, stem cell transplant and radiotherapy can also be used

CML

See Chronic leukaemia.

MULTIPLE MYELOMA

Multiple myeloma is a malignant disease characterised by proliferation of abnormal plasma cells producing immunoglobulins.

- Epidemiology: Age usually >60 years. 60–70 cases per million per year. Slightly more common in men than women

> The features of multiple myeloma can be remembered with the mnemonic **CRAB**: **C**alcium, **R**enal failure, **A**naemia, **B**one pain.

- Clinical presentation: Bone pain (back, ribs), pathological fracture, hypercalcaemia (confusion, constipation, thirst, polyuria), renal failure, amyloidosis (carpel tunnel syndrome), spinal cord compression, hyperviscosity
- Investigations:
  - Bedside: Bence-Jones protein in urine (mostly been superseded by serum free light chains)
  - Bloods: FBC (anaemia), ESR (↑), renal function (AKI), bone profile (↑Ca^{2+}), immunoglobulins, electrophoresis and serum free light chains
  - Imaging: X-ray (osteolytic lesions)
  - Arrange urgent hospital admission for people in whom investigations reveal moderate to severe hypercalcaemia (corrected calcium of 2.9 mmol/L or higher) or acute kidney injury
  - Arrange urgent referral to a haematologist (within 2 weeks) for further tests to confirm the diagnosis if serum and/or urine protein electrophoresis suggest myeloma
- Management:
  - Bisphosphonates for bone pain
  - Steroids (can help myeloma-induced hypercalcaemia)
  - Dialysis for renal failure
  - Plasmapheresis for hyperviscosity
  - Chemotherapy + bone marrow transplant

REFERENCES

National Institute for Health and Care Excellence. NICE Guidance 2015 for recognition and referral of haematological cancers.

https://cks.nice.org.uk/haematological-cancers-recognition-and-referral

National Institute for Health and Care Excellence. NICE Guidelines for when multiple myeloma is suspected. https://cks.nice.org.uk/multiple-myeloma

HAEMATOLOGY: QUESTIONS

ANAEMIA

1. How are anaemias classified?
2. What can cause a microcytic anaemia?
3. What is the most common cause of iron deficiency anaemia in men and postmenopausal women?
4. What can cause a macrocytic anaemia?
5. What blood results would be suggestive of a haemolytic anaemia?

HAEMATOLOGICAL MALIGNANCIES

1. How are leukaemias classified?
2. The Philadelphia chromosome is a translocation between which two chromosomes?
3. Which cell is classically found in affected lymph nodes of patients with Hodgkin's lymphoma?
4. Name the four myeloproliferative disorders.
5. Multiple myeloma is a proliferation of which immune cell?

CHAPTER 9

Infectious Diseases

9.1 HEPATITIS

DEFINITION

Hepatitis is defined as an inflammatory disease of the liver that can either be acute (<6 months) or chronic (>6 months). It can occur from a viral infection, autoimmune process, metabolic process or infiltrative diseases. Acute hepatitis has a variety of causes, whereas chronic hepatitis is most often due to viral infection (particularly hepatitis C and B).

EPIDEMIOLOGY

The most common cause of liver disease in the Western world is non-alcoholic fatty liver disease (NAFLD), of which steatohepatitis is the inflammatory stage of the condition. Hepatitis viruses (A–E) are the most common cause of hepatitis worldwide (Table 9.1.1). In the UK, the most common of these is hepatitis C virus, with an estimated prevalence of 200,000–500,000.

AETIOLOGY/PATHOLOGY

There are many causes of hepatitis:

Viral causes: Hepatitis A–E, cytomegalovirus, Epstein–Barr virus.

Autoimmune causes: Autoimmune hepatitis, primary biliary cirrhosis, primary sclerosing cholangitis.

Infiltrative causes: Sarcoidosis, Wilson's disease, hereditary haemochromatosis.

Metabolic causes: NAFLD, alcoholic liver disease, alpha-1-antitrypsin deficiency, drugs (e.g. methotrexate, amiodarone, isoniazid).

CLINICAL PRESENTATION

The clinical presentation of acute hepatitis may depend on the underlying cause. Generally, patients with hepatitis experience non-specific symptoms (fatigue, nausea, vomiting) followed by development of a fever, jaundice, RUQ discomfort and hepatomegaly. Chronic hepatitis presents with similar symptoms or symptoms of cirrhosis and liver failure (see Section 3.4).

EXAMINATION

Patients may have evidence of jaundice, lymphadenopathy, hepatomegaly and splenomegaly. Patients with chronic hepatitis may have evidence of cirrhosis and liver failure (see Section 3.4). There may be evidence of the underlying cause (e.g. IVDU marks suggestive of hepatitis B/C), obesity (NAFLD), Kayser–Fleischer rings (Wilson's disease), gynaecomastia, spider naevi (alcoholic liver disease).

INVESTIGATIONS

Bedside: Urinalysis (looking at bilirubin and urobilinogen).

Bloods: FBC (evidence of anaemia and thrombocytopenia), LFTs (evidence of hepatic disturbance), clotting (check liver synthetic function), U&Es (checking for hepatorenal syndrome), hepatitis viral serology, autoantibodies (smooth muscle antibodies [autoimmune hepatitis]), antimitochondrial antibodies (primary biliary cirrhosis), iron studies (haemochromatosis), ceruloplasmin (Wilson's disease), alpha-1-antitrypsin, immunoglobulins (IgA raised in alcoholic hepatitis, IgG raised in autoimmune hepatitis, IgM raised in primary biliary cirrhosis).

Imaging: USS liver.

MANAGEMENT

Management is dependent on the underlying cause.

Viral Hepatitis
Hepatitis A

Manifests as an acute hepatitis and is usually self-limiting with no long-term sequalae or carrier state.

Educate the patient about the condition, the need to avoid alcohol during the acute illness and for hygiene. Admission may be required if patients are severely unwell. **LFTs and prothrombin time** should be regularly measured. **Symptomatic treatment** should be given for nausea/pain or itch. The local health protection unit needs to be notified. Patients should avoid

Table 9.1.1 Types of viral hepatitis

Virus	DNA/RNA	Incubation period	Route	Notes
A	RNA	2 weeks	Fecal/Oral	IgM antibodies indicate recent infection IgG remains detectable lifelong
B	DNA	2–6 months	Parenteral	Source is usually from sexual contact or injecting drugs 10%–15% of chronic hepatitis
C	RNA	1–2 months	Parenteral	50%–80% of chronic hepatitis Risk of cirrhosis, HCC and end-stage liver disease
D	RNA		Parenteral	Needs hepatitis B in order for infection
E	RNA		Fecal/Oral	Dangerous in pregnancy

Table 9.1.2 Hepatitis B serology

HBsAg	Anti-HBc	Anti-HBs	Status
−	−	−	Susceptible to infection
−	+	+	Resolved infection
−	−	+	Vaccinated
+	+	−	Active HBV infection

going to work/school until they are no longer infectious (**7 days from jaundice/symptoms**). Contacts may be given hepatitis A vaccination if <1 week.

Hepatitis B

Incubation period for hepatitis B virus is 6–23 weeks and 10%–15% of infections manifest as chronic hepatitis B.

High risk groups include injecting drug users, multiple sexual partners, babies born to mothers who are carriers.

There are three major structural antigens: surface antigen (HBsAg), core antigen (HBcAg) and e antigen (HBeAg) (*Table 9.1.2*).

HBaAg is the first to appear and indicates active infection. If present >6 months, indicates carrier status. **Anti-HBc** (antibodies to core antigen) implies current or previous infection. **Anti-HBs** (antibodies to surface antigen) imply immunity (from either infection or vaccination).

Management includes educating the patient about the condition, the need to avoid alcohol during the acute illness and for hygiene. Admission may be required if patients are severely unwell. **LFTs and prothrombin time** should be regularly measured. **Symptomatic treatment** should be given for nausea/pain or itch. The local health protection unit needs to be notified. For chronic hepatitis B, NICE recommends using **PEGylated interferon-alpha** as first-line treatment.

Hepatitis C

Incubation period for hepatitis C is 2–25 weeks and 50%–80% of infections will develop into chronic hepatitis C.

Risk factors include injecting drug users, sexual transmission, unsterile tattoos, needlestick injuries and babies born to mothers who are carriers. Complications include **chronic hepatitis, cirrhosis, hepatocellular carcinoma (HCC) and liver failure**.

HCV RNA is the investigation of choice to diagnose acute HCV infection. Anti-HCV antibodies are detectable 3–4 months post-infection. Management includes educating the patient about the condition and the need to avoid alcohol during the acute illness in addition to lifestyle advice and informing injection/sexual contacts. Patients are given measures to prevent the spread of other blood-borne viruses and are offered hepatitis A+B vaccination. Medication depends of the viral genotype (at least six different ones are known). Treatment aims to reduce HCV RNA to undetectable levels 6 months following the end of treatment. Usually a combination of **protease inhibitors** (e.g. daclatasvir) with or without **ribavirin** are used. **Liver transplantation** is the treatment of choice for patients with end-stage liver disease. Regular alpha-fetoprotein measurement can be used to screen those with active hepatitis C to early identify transformation to HCC.

NON-ALCOHOLIC FATTY LIVER DISEASE

NAFLD describes a spectrum of progressive disease ranging from **steatosis** (fat in the liver) → steatohepatitis (fat with inflammation – known as **non-alcoholic steatohepatitis [NASH]**) → **fibrosis** → **cirrhosis** (see Section 3.4).

NASH is thought to have a prevalence of 3%–4% of the UK population. It is strongly associated with **obesity, hyperlipidaemia, type 2 diabetes** and **metabolic syndrome**. It is usually asymptomatic and is the most common cause for deranged LFTs in the UK. It should be suspected if a patient has risk factors for NAFLD (e.g. features of metabolic syndrome), persistent elevation of LFTs for ≥3 months and a USS liver showing fatty changes.

Management involves education, lifestyle advice about diet, weight loss and regular exercise and optimisation of management of associated conditions (diabetes, hypertension, hyperlipidaemia). Patients are monitored and assessed for cardiovascular risk. An **enhanced liver fibrosis** (**ELF**) test is used in individuals with NAFLD to test for advancement towards fibrosis.

AUTOIMMUNE HEPATITIS

Patients are classically **young females** with another **autoimmune** conditions. Can present with features of **acute hepatitis, amenorrhoea** or **chronic liver disease**. Investigations reveal a **raised antinuclear antibodies** (**sensitive**) and/or **anti-smooth muscle antibodies** (**specific**). Diagnosis is confirmed by **biopsy**. Medical management involves **immunosuppression** (e.g. steroids) or **liver transplantation**.

9.2 MENINGITIS

DEFINITION
Meningitis refers to inflammation of the meninges, which usually occurs secondary to infection.

EPIDEMIOLOGY
The incidence per year of acute bacterial meningitis in the UK is thought to be 2–5 per 100,000. It is one of the top 10 causes of infection-related death worldwide.

AETIOLOGY
Meningitis usually occurs secondary to infection, which may be bacterial (including mycobacteria), viral or fungal. Non-infectious causes include metastases, drugs (e.g. NSAIDs), sarcoidosis, SLE and vasculitis.

Bacterial meningitis occurs most commonly. The most common organisms by age group can be seen in *Table 9.2.1*.

The most common bacterial organisms include *Neisseria meningitidis* and *Streptococcus pneumoniae*. Less common bacterial organisms include *Haemophilus influenzae*, *Listeria monocytogenes* and TB.

Viral causes include enteroviruses, herpes simplex virus and cytomegalovirus.

Fungal meningitis usually occurs in immunocompromised patients and is most commonly caused by *Cryptococcus neoformans*.

PATHOLOGY
Infection can spread through a number of different routes to cause meningitis. The most common route of entry for bacterial meningitis is via haematogenous dissemination. When there is a septic shock response to meningococcus, this is termed meningococcal disease, which may occur with or without concurrent meningitis. The inflammatory response against the organism in the meninges causes oedema to accumulate, leading to raised intracranial pressure (ICP).

CLINICAL PRESENTATION
Non-specific symptoms include fever, anorexia, headache, muscle ache, nausea and vomiting.

Meningitis: Stiff neck and back, altered mental state, photophobia, bulging fontanelle in babies.

Advanced symptoms may include paresis, focal neurological deficit, seizures and coma.

EXAMINATION
Patients may have observations consistent with septic shock ($\downarrow$ BP, $\uparrow$ HR, $\uparrow$ temperature, $\uparrow$ capillary refill time).

If there is meningococcal septicaemia, then a non-blanching petechial rash may be seen.

Signs of meningitis include Kernig's sign (pain and resistance on passive knee extension with a fully flexed hip) and Brudzinski's sign (neck flexion causes flexion of hips and knees).

Signs of $\uparrow$ ICP (e.g. papilloedema, Cushing's reflex, see box) should prompt neurosurgical involvement.

Look for evidence of underlying causes for the meningitis (e.g. cold sores/genital vesicles [HSV]), lymphadenopathy, candidiasis (HIV), sore throat + jaundice + lymphadenopathy (EBV). It is important to perform otoscopy as meningitis can occur secondary to otitis media, which needs to be identified as ENT input will be required.

> ### Cushing's reflex
> Cushing's reflex is a physiological response to raised ICP. It results in a triad of raised BP, irregular breathing and bradycardia.

INVESTIGATIONS
Bedside: Ophthalmoscopy (looking for papilloedema) throat swabs, BM.

Bloods: FBC ($\downarrow$ WCC if immunocompromised), blood culture, lactate (septicaemia), viral serology (including HIV), whole blood PCR, inflammatory markers, blood gases, blood glucose.

Imaging: CXR (looking for signs of TB), CT (looking for $\uparrow$ ICP).

Invasive: LP (if no signs of $\uparrow$ ICP) with subsequent CSF cell count, glucose, protein, culture and Gram stain (*Table 9.2.2*). **Only perform LP if there are no signs of $\uparrow$ ICP.**

Table 9.2.1 Causative organisms of bacterial meningitis by age group

Age group	Causative organism
0–3 months	*Streptococcus agalactiae* (Group B streptococcus)
	Listeria monocytogenes
	Escherichia coli
3 months–6 years	*Neisseria meningitidis*
	S. pneumoniae
	Haemophilus influenzae
6 years–60 years	*N. meningitidis*
	S. pneumoniae
>60 years	*S. pneumoniae*
	N. meningitidis
	L. monocytogenes
Immunocompromised patients	*L. monocytogenes*

Table 9.2.2 CSF findings in meningitis

	Appearance	Glucose	Protein	White cells
Bacterial	Cloudy	↓↓ (1/2 plasma)	↑	↑ Polymorphs
Viral	Clear	Normal	Normal/↑	↑ Lymphocytes
Tuberculosis	Cloudy	↓↓	↑	↑ Lymphocytes

DIFFERENTIAL DIAGNOSIS

The differential diagnosis for meningitis includes encephalitis, brain abscess, septicaemia, subarachnoid haemorrhage and infectious diseases such as tetanus, dengue fever and malaria. A travel history is important.

MANAGEMENT

Adult acute

Patients should be resuscitated via an ABCDE approach and managed in ITU if septic or have ↑ ICP.

For suspected meningococcal disease in the community (meningitis with non-blanching rash or meningococcal septicaemia) – give **benzylpenicillin** at the earliest opportunity (IM/IV) unless there is a clear anaphylaxis history.

Local policies vary for additional antibiotic therapy but usually involve adding a broad-spectrum IV antibiotic (such as **cefotaxime**) and IV **dexamethasone**. If a patient has suspected viral meningitis, IV **acyclovir** is widely used but there is no evidence to support its use.

If the patient does not have ↑ ICP or signs of shock, then perform an LP. If an organism has been isolated, seek microbiology help on further management.

Patients should be carefully monitored for signs of airway compromise and hypovolaemia and for complications of meningitis. These include:

- Hydrocephalus
- Seizures
- Hearing loss
- Brain abscess

Subsequent management

Meningitis is a notifiable disease and you should contact your local Public Health England Health Protection Unit for all cases of probable or confirmed meningitis. Depending on the suspected or confirmed causative agent, contact tracing and prophylaxis may be necessary. Guidance is available at the time of reporting to Public Health England.

> **Microbiology tips**
>
> Common phrases to describe causative organisms in meningitis:
>
> - Gram-positive cocci = *Streptococcus pneumoniae*
> - Gram-negative diplococci = *Neisseria meningitidis*
> - Gram-positive anaerobic bacilli = *Listeria monocytogenes*
> - Gram-negative facultative anaerobic bacilli = *Escherichia coli*
> - Gram-negative coccobacilli = *Haemophilus influenzae*

9.3 HUMAN IMMUNODEFICIENCY VIRUS

DEFINITION

The human immunodeficiency virus (HIV) is an RNA retrovirus that infects cells of the immune system.

There are two variants: HIV-1 (more common in the UK) and HIV-2 (more common in west Africa).

EPIDEMIOLOGY

Around 35 million people worldwide are infected with HIV. The vast majority of these cases are in Africa.

In the UK, around 100,000 people have HIV with 1 in 4 unaware of their infection. It is most prevalent among men who have sex with men and black-African heterosexual men and women. Other risk factors include multiple sexual partners, a history of STIs, hepatitis B or C, occupational exposure (e.g. needlestick injury), previous transfusions of blood products (especially those given prior to HIV screening) and transfusions and transplants in countries without screening for HIV.

AETIOLOGY

HIV is an RNA retrovirus that infects people from sexual contact with infected persons, contact with infected blood and blood products, IV drug use or vertical (mother/child) transmission. The HIV virus is a spherical-shaped virus that contains two copies of single-stranded RNA surrounded by capsid of viral protein (p24). The capsid also contains the three enzymes that are important in HIV, which can be remembered by the mnemonic **RIP**: **R**everse transcriptase, **I**ntegrase and **P**rotease. Surrounding the capsid is a viral envelope containing glycoproteins that bind to immune cells (such as gp120). Some of these glycoproteins (gp120) have a variable antigenic region, so once the immune system has developed antibodies against it, it can change. This is why we cannot vaccinate against HIV.

PATHOLOGY

Once the virus has been introduced into the bloodstream it replicates and binds to immune cells:

- Surface glycoproteins bind to receptors (such as CD4+ and CCR5) of immune cells
- The viral envelope and cell membrane of the immune cells fuse together, allowing entry of the virus
- Once inside the cell, **reverse transcriptase** is released and converts the HIV RNA into HIV DNA, allowing entry of the DNA to enter the cell nucleus of the immune cell (e.g. CD4 cell)
- Once HIV DNA is inside the nucleus, the enzyme **integrase** integrates HIV DNA with host cell DNA
- Now that HIV DNA is integrated into the host cell DNA, the DNA is replicated and more HIV proteins and RNA are made, which are initially assembled as long-chain molecules and are non-infectious

- These newly formed non-infectious molecules are released by the host cell and react with the enzyme **protease**, which acts to splice the long chain non-infectious molecule into shorter-chain molecules that combine to form an infectious form of HIV.

Because of how important these enzymes are in the development of HIV, they are targets of drug therapy.

Nucleoside reverse transcriptase inhibitors (NRTIs) and non-nucleoside reverse transcriptase inhibitors (NNRTIs) target reverse transcriptase. Integrase inhibitors target integrase and protease inhibitors target protease. There are also therapies that aim to prevent the fusion of HIV to immune cells (fusion inhibitors).

CLINICAL PRESENTATION

There are a number of stages of HIV infection and patients may present at different stages of the infection.

Acute infection (<2 weeks) is often asymptomatic. **Acute retroviral syndrome** (when seroconversion happens) occurs 2–6 weeks after exposure and has symptoms similar to glandular fever (e.g. malaise, fever, sore throat, lymphadenopathy, diarrhoea) and may include a maculopapular rash. Following seroconversion, patients can be asymptomatic for a long period of time or develop **persistent generalised lymphadenopathy** until constitutional symptoms develop, which include pyrexia, night sweats and weight loss. Patients may then start to develop recurrent infections (e.g. candidiasis, seborrhoeic dermatitis). Following a long period of time with HIV infection (approximately 10 years), patients may develop **acquired immunodeficiency syndrome** (**AIDS**) (defined as a CD4 count <200 cells/μL) and may present with a series of AIDS-defining conditions (see box).

EXAMINATION

Signs on examination vary depending on how long a patient has had the virus for. If a patient presents with an acute retroviral syndrome then a maculopapular rash may be found in addition to lymphadenopathy (including inguinal). Other signs may be non-specific and include mouth ulceration or signs of infection (e.g. candida). Patients may have signs on examination from AIDs-defining conditions.

Complications of HIV (bold are AIDS-defining illnesses)

Recurrent infections (e.g. recurrent **pneumonia**)

Respiratory: ***Pneumocystis jiroveci*** pneumonia, Cryptococcus, **tuberculosis**

Neurological: **Cerebral toxoplasmosis, cryptococcal meningitis, primary CNS lymphoma** (associated with EBV), **encephalitis (CMV/HIV), progressive multifocal leukoencephalopathy (PML), AIDS dementia complex**

Gastrointestinal: Candidiasis, diarrhoea (HIV itself, bacterial infection, protozoa [**cryptosporidium**])

Skin: **Kaposi sarcoma** (caused by human herpes virus 8)

Eye: **CMV retinitis** (ophthalmoscopy classically shows 'mozzarella pizza' sign).

Cancer: **non-Hodgkin's lymphoma, Burkitt's lymphoma**

Psychology: Depression

INVESTIGATIONS

The first-line investigations for HIV are the combined HIV antibody and p24 antigen tests. This '*fourth* generation' test has a *four*-week window period, which detects the majority of people infected with HIV. A positive test requires a second test for confirmation, whereas a negative test requires a repeat after 12 weeks.

There are additional point-of-care tests (e.g. finger-prick or mouth swabs) used in genital-urinary medicine (GUM) clinics that can also be used but are more likely to give a false positive result. These tests have a 12-week window.

Bedside: Finger-prick HIV test, ophthalmoscopy (if suspecting CMV retinitis).

Bloods: HIV antibody and p24 antigen tests (diagnostic), LFTs (often deranged), FBC (neutropenia, anaemia, thrombocytopenia), viral load, CD4 count, resistance profile.

Imaging: CXR (if suspected TB or *Pneumocystis jirovecii* infection).

DIFFERENTIAL DIAGNOSIS

HIV can manifest in a multitude of signs and symptoms. For the primary HIV infection, the differential includes glandular fever, toxoplasmosis, rubella, viral hepatitis (see Section 9.1), herpes simplex infection, syphilis and influenza.

MANAGEMENT

Patients with no need for urgent admission (e.g. acutely unwell, respiratory infection, CMV retinitis, neurological complications such as meningitis) should be referred to a GUM clinic or HIV specialist within 2 weeks of diagnosis.

Chronic disease
Non-pharmacological

- Educate about HIV
- Promote safer sexual practice if there is a risk through sexual contact, and direct people who inject drugs to local services

- Patients with a new diagnosis of HIV should be tested for past or present infections, including tuberculosis, toxoplasmosis, CMV, hepatitis B/C and syphili
- HIV testing for sexual partners
- HIV monitoring including CD4 count and viral load
- HIV predisposes to a number of conditions, so monitoring for the following is needed:
  - Cardiovascular disease (lipids)
  - Cervical cancer (yearly smears)
  - Infections including vaccinations for influenza, pneumococcal, hepatitis A, B, tetanus, diphtheria and polio

Pharmacological

- The British HIV Association recommends that therapy-naive patients should be started on two nucleoside reverse transcriptase inhibitors (NRTIs) (e.g. tenofovir-DF and emtricitabine) plus one of the following:
  - Ritonavir-boosted protease inhibitor
  - Non-nucleoside reverse transcriptase inhibitor
  - Integrase inhibitor (e.g. raltegravir)

Post-exposure prophylaxis after sexual exposure (PEPSE)

PEPSE is an emergency method of HIV prevention and is recommended when there is a significant risk of HIV transmission. It is not recommended if there is sexual contact with an HIV+ source who is on medication with a confirmed and sustained (>6 months) viral load. PEPSE can be offered up to 72 hours post-exposure, ideally within the first 24 hours.

The first-line regime is two NRTIs (tenofovir DF and emtricitabine) and an integrase inhibitor (raltegravir) for 28 days.

Blood tests are taken at baseline and 8–12 weeks post-exposure.

Pre-exposure prophylaxis (PrEP)

Recent trials have demonstrated that PrEP, in the form of two NRTIs (tenofovir-DF and emtricitabine), given in addition to condoms and risk-reduction counselling prior to sexual contact reduces the relative risk of acquiring HIV compared with placebo or no prophylaxis.

These trials looked at transmission in either HIV-negative men or transgender women who have sex with men, or HIV-negative individuals in a heterosexual partnership with a person already infected with HIV.

Patients must be HIV negative prior to starting.

PrEP is currently undergoing clinical trials in England and Wales.

9.4 SEXUALLY TRANSMITTED INFECTIONS

DEFINITION

Sexually transmitted infections (STIs) are infections that are transmitted from person to person via sexual contact. There are a number of STIs to be aware of for your medical school finals that include chlamydia, gonorrhoea, syphilis, trichomonas, genital herpes, genital warts and HIV (see Section 9.3).

TREATING STIS

Patients should ideally be referred to genital-urinary medicine (GUM) clinics for treatment of STIs. Here, specialists can take a thorough sexual history, screen for other STIs, provide education, contact tracing and partner notification. Generally speaking, sexual intercourse (genital, oral and anal) even with a condom, should be avoided until completion of treatment of both the patient and partner (if infected).

Risk factors for STIs include age <25 years, new sexual partner, ≥1 sexual partner in last year and not using condoms.

CHLAMYDIA

Chlamydia (*Chlamydia trachomatis)* is the most common bacterial STI in the UK, which generally infects the urethra in men and vagina women but can also affect the endocervix (women), conjunctiva, rectum and nasopharynx. Chlamydia is a gram-negative organism and causes an infection that has the potential to ascend (and cause complications – see later), by which point it is called a complicated chlamydia infection. Approximately 1.5%−10% of individuals aged 15–24 have chlamydia, with approximately 200,000 new diagnoses each year reported.

Clinical presentation

The condition is may be asymptomatic (70% women, 50% men). If symptomatic, presentations include:

Women: Vaginal discharge, PV bleeding (post-coital/intermenstrual), dysuria or complications.

Men: Urethritis, dysuria or urethral discharge.

Investigations

First-catch urine sample or swab (endocervical/vulvovaginal in women) can be sent for nucleic acid amplification testing (NAAT).

Management

Treatment should be initiated in all people who test positive for chlamydia or have signs or symptoms strongly suggestive for chlamydia (following testing for other STIs).

Pharmacological options include azithromycin (1 g single dose) or doxycycline (100 mg BD for 7 days). If **azithromycin** taken (single dose), then abstinence from sexual activity is advised for 7 days. If breast-feeding/pregnant, doxycycline is contraindicated; however, azithromycin can still be used. A test of cure is recommended for chlamydia in pregnancy 6 weeks post-treatment.

Complications

Women: Pelvic inflammatory disease (PID), endometritis, salpingitis, infertility, perihepatitis (Fitz-Hugh–Curtis syndrome), ectopic pregnancy, reactive arthritis.

Men: Epididymo-orchitis, reactive arthritis.

Important to know: There is a National Chlamydia Screening Programme in the UK that recommends annual screening of sexually active people under the age of 25 (or more often if the patient has many partners).

GONORRHOEA

Gonorrhoea (*Neisseria gonorrhoeae*) is a common bacterial STI in the UK that affects the urethra, endocervix, conjunctiva, rectum and pharynx. Gonorrhoea is a gram-negative intracellular diplococcus.

Clinical presentation

Women: Gonorrhoea may be asymptomatic in 50% of women or cause symptoms such as dysuria or increased/altered vaginal discharge generally <10 days post-exposure.

Men: Gonorrhoea is usually symptomatic (unless rectal/pharyngeal infection) causing urethral discharge or dysuria usually 2–5 days after exposure.

Investigations

First-catch urine sample or swab (endocervical/vulvo-vaginal in women) can be sent for NAAT and MC + S to confirm diagnosis. If symptomatic or suspicious of gonorrhoea, a swab for culture should be taken from the affected site as well as NAAT testing due to emerging antibiotic resistance.

Management

For a confirmed or suspected uncomplicated anogenital or pharyngeal infection, a combination of IM **ceftriaxone** and oral **azithromycin** is recommended. **A test of cure is recommended** and follow-up is recommended 2 weeks after treatment to confirm resolution of symptoms, eradication of the organism, confirm partner notification and reinforce safe sexual practice. Different treatment regimes are required if patients have PID/epididymo-orchitis or conjunctivitis secondary to gonorrhoea. If patients have disseminated gonorrhoea (see later), then hospital admission is advised for IV antibiotics.

Complications

Gonorrhoea can have a number of complications, such as epididymitis, infertility and prostatitis in men and PID and spontaneous abortions in women.

Disseminated gonorrhoea infection may occur following haematogenous dissemination resulting in skin lesions, arthralgia and arthritis.

For both gonorrhoea and chlamydia: vulvovaginal swabbing is superior to urine sampling in women.

TRICHOMONAS VAGINALIS

Trichomonas vaginalis (TV) is a flagellated protozoon STI that classically affects the urethra in both sexes and the vagina in women.

Clinical presentation

Up to half of men and women are asymptomatic with TV infection.

Women: Typical symptoms include mucopurulent, yellow, odorous vaginal discharge. Vulval itching and dysuria may be present. A classic finding is a 'strawberry cervix', although this is only found in around 2% of patients.

Men: Urethral discharge and/or dysuria.

Investigations

Women: A **high vaginal swab** (from the posterior fornix) should be taken for MC + S.

Men: First-catch urine to be sent for MC + S. A urethral swab can also be taken. Live protozoa can also be seen on a microscope slide in GUM services with access to microscopy.

Management

For symptomatic patients with confirmed TV, **metronidazole** is the recommended antibiotic. Contact tracing and treatment of partners is recommended. Test of cure is recommended for TV in pregnancy.

Complications

TV may be associated with perinatal complications in pregnant women (such as preterm delivery and low birth weight).

SYPHILIS

Syphilis is an STI caused by the spirochaete bacterium *Treponema pallidum.* If left untreated, syphilis can progress through distinct disease stages: primary, secondary, latent and tertiary disease.

Transmission of syphilis can be via direct contact with an infectious lesion, bodily fluids from an infected person or by vertical transmission during pregnancy. In the UK, syphilis is predominantly found in white men aged 25–34 years who have sex with men.

Clinical presentation

Syphilis can present at various stages along its clinical course if left untreated:

Primary syphilis: Following an incubation period of approximately 9–90 days, the signs of primary syphilis may become apparent. These include the development of chancres (painless genital ulcers) that typically resolve spontaneously even without treatment.

Secondary syphilis: Approximately 25% of patients with primary syphilis will go on to the secondary stage. Hallmarks of secondary syphilis appear 4–10 weeks after the chancres and include:

- Skin manifestations: Widespread mucocutaneous rash
- Lymphadenopathy, commonly inguinal and cervical
- Condylomata lata (wart-like lesions on genitals)
- Neurological manifestations: Meningitis, cranial nerve palsies, optic neuropathy, uveitis
- Systemic manifestations: Hepatitis, glomerulonephritis, splenomegaly

Latent disease: Approximately 3–12 weeks following secondary syphilis, the disease will enter a latent stage where patients are completely asymptomatic. One-quarter of these patients may experience a recurrence of secondary disease. Latent disease is classified into two stages: early latent syphilis, where an individual has been infected for less than 2 years, and late latent syphilis, where infection has been present for over 2 years.

Tertiary syphilis: Occurs in approximately one-third of untreated patients 20–40 years after the initial infection. Clinical manifestations are divided into cardiovascular, neurological and gummatous:

- Cardiovascular: Aortitis, aortic regurgitation, heart failure, angina, aneurysm
- Neurological: Spectrum of involvement including asymptomatic changes in CSF to meningovascular inflammation, memory loss, psychosis and inflammation of the spinal column causing paraesthesia, areflexia, ataxia, optic atrophy and an Argyll Robertson pupil (where the **a**ccommodation **r**eflex is **p**reserved but there is loss of the light reflex)
- Gummatous: Granulomatous lesions with a necrotic centre that most commonly occur in the liver, nervous system, skin and bones

Investigations

Dark ground microscopy of lesions and polymerase chain reaction (PCR) swabs can help demonstrate *T. pallidum* from lesions. Blood tests can also be used for screening and effects of treatment. An enzyme immunoassay (EIA) antibody test is performed first. If this is negative, testing stops and a negative result is reported. If positive, the EIA will be repeated. If still positive, a second treponemal test, either treponemal pallidum particle agglutination test (TPPA)/treponemal pallidum haemagglutination assay or VDRL will be performed giving a quantitative result, which is then backed up by a rapid plasma reagin (RPR) test that gives the quantitative result. IgM testing can also be useful to determine recent infection.

Once infected, EIA antibody testing for syphilis will always remain positive; however, the RPR is used to determine active infection, whether treatment has been effective, and to assess reinfection.

Management

Pharmacological options differ depending on the clinical stage. For 'early' syphilis (primary, secondary or early latent) one dose of benzathine penicillin G is recommended. Late latent and tertiary syphilis requires once weekly doses of benzathine penicillin G for 3 weeks. Tertiary syphilis requires a longer course of benzathine. For neurosyphilis, corticosteroids (to reduce inflammation) are given alongside 14 days of IM procaine penicillin and probenecid (to protect the kidneys).

Treatment of syphilis is associated with a Jarisch–Herxheimer reaction (febrile illness) from endotoxin release.

Patients should be followed up and have repeat RPR/TPPA or VDRL titres taken to check whether treatment was successful.

GENITAL HERPES

Genital herpes is a viral STI caused by herpes simplex virus (HSV) following direct contact with lesions. Lesions can appear anywhere on the skin, but most commonly occur on the lips or genitals.

Clinical presentation

Primary infection presents with painful genital ulcers with erythema and tender inguinal lymphadenitis usually <1 week post-exposure. Lesions crust over initially, then heal. Discharge may also occur.

Investigations

Swabs from infected lesions (anogenital/rectal) are sent for PCR/NAAT. HSV serology can also assess whether this is the first exposure to the virus, which is useful in pregnancy.

Management

Non-pharmacological management includes saline bathing, analgesia, topical anaesthetic agents. Acyclovir is used if presentation <5 days. Barrier methods of contraception should be used to decrease transmission risk. For people presenting with more than six outbreaks per year (more common is HSV2), then suppressive acyclovir can be used on a daily basis.

Considerable psychological morbidity is associated with genital HSV infection, with some patients requiring extensive support and counselling.

INFECTIOUS DISEASES: QUESTIONS

9.1 HEPATITIS

1. Name three causes of hepatitis.
2. Which viral hepatitis can lead to chronic liver failure?
3. What would the immunological profile of a patient who has a resolved hepatitis B infection look like?

9.2 MENINGITIS

1. What features of CSF analysis are suggestive of bacterial meningitis?
2. A 22-year-old man presents with symptoms of meningitis. CSF isolates a gram-negative diplococcus. What is the causative organism?

9.3 HIV

1. What are the symptoms of acute retroviral syndrome?
2. Which tests are considered first-line to diagnose HIV? What are the 'window periods'?
3. Name three complications of HIV infection.
4. How long post-exposure can PEPSE medications be given?
5. Which classes of medications are given to patients with a new diagnosis of HIV?

9.4 SEXUALLY TRANSMITTED INFECTIONS

1. Match the condition to the correct organism description.

Condition:

Trichomonas vaginalis

Chlamydia

Syphilis

Gonorrhoea

Genital herpes

Organism:

Virus

Gram-negative diplococci

Gram-negative organism

Spirochaete

Protozoon

2. Name three complications of untreated chlamydia infection.
3. What are the management options for a patient with an uncomplicated anogenital gonorrhoea infection?
4. Describe the stages of an untreated syphilis infection.
5. How does a genital ulcer caused by genital herpes differ from an ulcer caused by primary syphilis?

CHAPTER **10**

Dermatology

10.1 ECZEMA

DEFINITION

Eczema is chronic, inflammatory skin condition characterised by papules and vesicles on an erythematous base.

EPIDEMIOLOGY

Atopic eczema is the most common type of eczema. Around 80% of cases of atopic eczema occur before 5 years of age.

AETIOLOGY

The aetiology of eczema is not fully understood but factors such as genetic predisposition, dysfunction of the skin barrier and immune system dysfunction are thought to play a part. Exacerbating factors include environmental triggers (allergens), infections and heat. Other atopic conditions are often present (asthma, allergic rhinitis).

CLINICAL PRESENTATION

Atopic eczema typically presents as an intense, itchy, erythematous rash on the flexure surfaces, sparing the groin and axillary regions. The rash typically starts in childhood and is episodic in nature. The clinical presentation varies from mild to severe.

EXAMINATION

The distribution of the rash may vary based on the age of the patient. Typically, in adults there is generalised dryness and itching.

Acute lesions appear erythematous and vesicular and may potentially weep. Eczema may become infected without systemic infection. Chronic eczema lesions can be identified by excoriation marks and lichenification (thickened skin from chronic scratching).

INVESTIGATIONS

Atopic eczema is primarily a clinical diagnosis and investigations are often not required. If lesions look infected, then temperature can be measured to look for the degree of systemic infection.

NICE diagnostic criteria states that atopic eczema is likely if the following are fulfilled:

An itchy skin condition (or parental report of scratching) plus **three or more of the following**:

- Visible flexural dermatitis involving the skin creases, such as the bends of the elbows or behind the knees (or visible eczema on the cheeks and/or extensor areas in children aged 18 months or younger)
- Personal history of flexural eczema (or eczema on the cheeks and/or extensor areas in children aged 18 months or younger)
- Personal history of dry skin in the last 12 months

- Personal history of asthma or allergic rhinitis (or history of atopic disease in a first-degree relative of a child aged under 4 years)
- Onset of signs and symptoms before the age of 2 years (this criterion should not be used in children younger than 4 years of age)

DIFFERENTIAL DIAGNOSIS

The differential diagnosis of atopic eczema includes psoriasis, allergic contact dermatitis, seborrhoeic dermatitis or a skin infection (e.g. fungal, scabies).

MANAGEMENT

The management of eczema is guided by the severity of the disease. NICE categorise eczema as:

- Mild: Dry skin with infrequent itching
- Moderate: Dry skin + frequent itching + redness
- Severe: Widespread dry skin + incessant itching + redness
- Infected: Eczema that shows evidence of weeping, crusting or pustules, with fever or malaise

Tools for assessing severity include the patient-oriented eczema measure (POEM).

Chronic disease

Non-pharmacological

- Education about the condition to patient and parents (if the patient is a child)
- Identification and avoidance of exacerbating factors

Pharmacological

The mainstay of eczema treatment involves emollients:

- Encourage frequent and regular usage of emollients (underuse may increase flares)
- For flares, increase emollient usage and consider topical corticosteroids and antihistamines
- A short course of oral corticosteroids can be considered for severe eczema flares in adults
- Antihistamines: If there is severe itch or urticaria, a non-sedating antihistamine can be prescribed (e.g. cetirizine, fexofenadine)

The following treatments can be initiated in secondary care by a dermatologist:

- Calcineurin inhibitors (e.g. tacrolimus, pimecrolimus)
- UVB light treatment
- Systemic treatment for severe eczema, e.g. azathioprine, mycophenolate mofetil
- Biologics (e.g. dupilumab)

COMPLICATIONS OF ATOPIC ECZEMA

- Lichenification: Thickening of the skin as a result of chronic scratching of the skin
- Infection:
  - Eczema may become infected with **Staphylococcus aureus** with worsening redness of the skin, crusting and weeping of lesions. Treatment includes topical flucloxacillin if localised or oral if extensive areas of infection (unless allergic, in which case clarithromycin is given)
  - Herpes simplex infection (**eczema herpeticum**) should be considered whenever there are widespread vesicular lesions that coalesce into large bleeding areas. Patients may have fever and lymphadenopathy. This is a medical emergency and should be managed in hospital
  - Superficial **fungal infections** may also occur in patients with atopic eczema
- Psychosocial problems: Atopic eczema can cause distress for patients and it can be a particular problem during childhood and adolescence, where it may be associated with behavioural problems and depression

REFERENCE

National Institute for Health and Care Excellence. NICE Eczema – atopic. https://cks.nice.org.uk/eczema-atopic

10.2 PSORIASIS

DEFINITION
Psoriasis is a chronic, systemic, inflammatory skin condition that typically takes a relapsing-remitting course.

EPIDEMIOLOGY
Psoriasis affects approximately 2% of the UK population.

AETIOLOGY
The cause of psoriasis is not known; however, there are a number of factors associated with its onset and exacerbations that can be divided into environmental, genetic and immunological:

Genetic: There is a strong hereditary component to psoriasis (30%–40% have a family history) and a number of different genetic loci have been identified to contribute (e.g. psoriasis susceptibility 1–9 [PSORS1-9]).

Immunological: There is evidence that psoriasis has an autoimmune component with T cells releasing cytokines, causing symptoms of the disease. This could explain why immunological therapies are effective.

Environmental: Trauma (Koebner phenomenon), stress, smoking, alcohol, infection, corticosteroid withdrawal and hormonal changes. Psoriasis may be associated with other conditions, such as psoriatic arthropathy, inflammatory bowel disease (particularly Crohn's disease), metabolic syndrome and depression.

PATHOLOGY
There is hyperproliferation of keratinocytes and inflammatory cell infiltration of the skin.

There are different types of psoriasis (*Table 10.2.1*). The most common type is chronic plaque psoriasis (85%), followed by localised pustular psoriasis that affects the palms and soles. Others forms of psoriasis include guttate psoriasis (post-streptococcal infection) and nail psoriasis.

CLINICAL PRESENTATION
Patients classically present with well-demarcated raised erythematous scaly plaques on the extensor surfaces and scalp. These lesions can occasionally be itchy or painful.

Fifty percent of patients have associated nail changes (pitting, onycholysis, subungual hyperkeratosis). Ten percent of patients also have psoriatic arthropathy, and this can present as arthritis of the small joints of the hands/feet, similar to RA.

EXAMINATION
The key to examining for psoriasis is to not just examine where a rash is presented to you but to examine all areas where there may be a rash. This includes scalp and all extensor surfaces.

Table 10.2.1 Types of psoriasis

Type	Features
Chronic plaque	Most common form. Well-demarcated raised plaques involving the extensor surfaces (knees, elbows), scalp, hair or sacrum
Localised pustular	Yellow/brown sterile pustules on the palms or soles
Scalp	Similar to dandruff but with thicker scale
Flexure	Typically affects the axilla and submammary area. Plaques are smoother and appear glazed
Guttate	Classically occurs poststreptococcal throat infection. Presents with symmetrical circular lesions on the trunk and limbs
Nail	Can present with any sign (pitting, onycholysis [loosening or separation of a fingernail or toenail from its nail bed], subungual hyperkeratosis) Have to differentiate from fungal nail infection
Erythroderma	Intense and widespread reddening of the skin affecting 90% or more of the skin surface Medical emergency
Generalised pustular	Multiple yellow/brown pustules on an erythematous base and spread rapidly. Needs hospital treatment

Usually there will be multiple, well-demarcated raised erythematous plaques on extensor surfaces. Comment on their size and any scaling present.

Remember to examine the nails for associated changes of pitting, subungual hyperkeratosis and onycholysis.

For completeness, perform a joint examination on the hand and wrist looking for a symmetrical polyarthropathy or signs of an active synovitis that could be consistent with psoriatic arthritis.

DIFFERENTIAL DIAGNOSIS
The differential diagnosis for psoriasis includes eczema, seborrhoeic dermatitis, fungal skin infection, cellulitis, secondary syphilis, lichen planus and discoid lupus erythematosus. Guttate psoriasis may present similarly to pityriasis rosea.

MANAGEMENT
Chronic disease
Non-pharmacological
- Educate about the condition
- Provide lifestyle advice to reduce the risk of exacerbations (smoking cessation, weight loss, alcohol advice)

- Assess for anxiety/depression
- Advise to seek medical attention if they experience unexplained joint pain or swelling (psoriatic arthritis)
- Assess the patient's cardiovascular risk every 5 years (↑ risk of cardiovascular disease, VTE and metabolic syndrome); check lipids, glucose and BP

Pharmacological

- Regular emollients may help to reduce scale loss + pruritus
- First-line: NICE recommend a **potent corticosteroid** applied once daily plus **vitamin D analogue** applied **once daily** (applied separately, one in the morning and the other in the evening) for up to 4 weeks as initial treatment
- Second-line: If no improvement after 8 weeks, then offer a **vitamin D analogue twice daily**
- Third-line: If no improvement after 8–12 weeks, then offer either a **potent corticosteroid** applied **twice daily** for up to 4 weeks or a **coal tar preparation** (dithranol) applied once or twice daily

- Other options include:
  - Topical retinoids
  - Salicylic acid

Secondary care options

- Narrow band ultraviolet B light three times a week
- Photochemotherapy is also used: Psoralen + ultraviolet A light (PUVA)
- Methotrexate (especially if associated joint disease)
- Ciclosporin (leads to quick remissions, temporary measure)
- Acitretin (systemic retinoid)
- Biologics (infliximab, etanercept, adalimumab)

REFERENCE

National Institute for Health and Care Excellence. NICE Guidelines Psoriasis. https://cks.nice.org.uk/psoriasis

10.3 SKIN CANCER

BASAL CELL CARCINOMA
Definition
Basal cell carcinoma (BCC) is cancer derived from the basal cells of the epidermis.

Epidemiology
BCC is the most common form of skin cancer in the Western world with approximately 75,000 diagnosed each year in the UK.

Aetiology/Pathology
A number of factors are thought to play a role in the development of BCCs:

- UV radiation: Both cumulative lifetime exposure and intense exposure predisposes to BCCs
- Immunosuppression (e.g. post-organ transplantation)
- Genetics (loss of function of the PTCH gene and genetic syndromes such as Gorlin's syndrome)

Clinical presentation
As BCCs are more likely to occur with UV radiation, they usually appear on sun-exposed areas (head/neck) which is where patients often notice them, although they can occur anywhere. Lesions are painless but may bleed if they are traumatised. They can be locally destructive if they enlarge. Metastatic potential is extremely low, ranging between 0.0028 and 0.55 of all BCC cases.

Examination
The most common type of BCCs is a nodular BCC (known as a 'rodent ulcer') that present as a papule or nodule with surface telangiectasia, which may ulcerate in the centre.

Investigations
An incisional or punch biopsy from the lesion may be used to confirm the diagnosis.

Management
Management largely depends on the risk. Lesions are classified as either high risk (see box) or low risk (if there are no features of high risk).

NICE guidelines recommend referring patients down the suspected skin cancer referral pathway for an appointment within 2 weeks only in cases of high-risk BCC.

There are a number of options for treating low-risk BCCs:

- Topical 5-flurouracil and imiquimod cream
- Cryotherapy
- Curettage and cautery
- Radiotherapy (also could be a first-line treatment in elderly and/or inoperable cases)
- Photodynamic therapy

High-risk BCC requires surgical excision with predetermined clinical margins or Mohs micrographic surgery.

> **High-risk BCC**
>
> Patient <24 years old
>
> Immunocompromised
>
> Genetic predisposition
>
> Recurrent/incompletely treated BCC
>
> Lesions on nose or lips
>
> Lesions >2 cm in diameter below the clavicle or >1 cm above the clavicle
>
> Poorly defined margins
>
> Lesions over important anatomical structures
>
> Histological subtypes: Morphoeic, micronodular, infiltrative, basosquamous

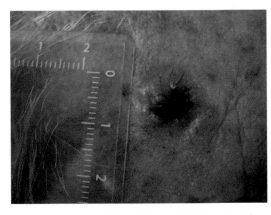

Figure 10.3.1 Nodular and ulcerated BCC on the right forehead. Very slowly growing, approximately 2-year history. Examination reveals pearly nodule with telangiectasias and haemorrhagic crust (feature of ulceration).

SQUAMOUS CELL CARCINOMA
Definition
Squamous cell carcinoma (SCC) is malignant tumour of keratinocytes found in the epidermis and stratified squamous mucosa. SCC may give rise to local metastases or spread to local lymph nodes.

Epidemiology
SCC is the second most common type of skin cancer in the Western world with approximately 25,000 SCCs diagnosed every year in the UK.

Aetiology/Pathology

A number of factors are thought to play a role in the development of SCCs:

- UV radiation: Cumulative lifetime exposure is a major risk factor; this leads to defective DNA replication and transcription in keratinocytes
- HPV has been associated with the development of certain types of SCC
- Premalignant conditions such as Bowen's disease or actinic keratosis

Clinical presentation

Similar to BCCs, SCCs occur on sun-exposed areas (e.g. head/neck/dorsal aspect of hands and lower legs) and this is where patients are likely to notice them, although they can occur anywhere. There is usually a long history as lesions are slow growing.

Examination

Examination may reveal a keratotic papule or plaque that may have a crusted or scaly surface. Regional lymph nodes should also be examined for local metastases.

Investigations

An incisional biopsy from the lesion can be used to confirm the diagnosis.

Differential diagnosis

The main differential diagnosis for SCCs is a keratoacanthoma – a rapidly enlarging nodule with a keratin centre. The main difference between a keratoacanthoma and a SCC is the time it takes for the lesion to develop. SCCs are much slower to develop than a keratoacanthoma, which will spontaneously involute.

Management

NICE guidelines recommend referring patients down the suspected skin cancer referral pathway for an appointment within 2 weeks.

SCCs are usually managed with surgical excision. Curettage and cautery can be used for smaller or low-risk tumours. Radiotherapy can be used if surgery is not a feasible option or as an adjuvant treatment for high-risk SCCs. High-risk SCCs include those whose depth/invasion >2 mm, located on the ear or lip or poorly differentiated on histology.

MALIGNANT MELANOMA

Definition

Malignant melanoma is a skin cancer resulting from melanocytes in the basal layer of the epidermis. It is considered to be the most serious form of skin cancer. Melanoma can arise from otherwise normal-appearing skin (in about 75% of melanomas) or from within a mole or freckle, which starts to grow larger and change in appearance.

Epidemiology

Around 13,000 malignant melanomas of the skin are diagnosed each year in the UK.

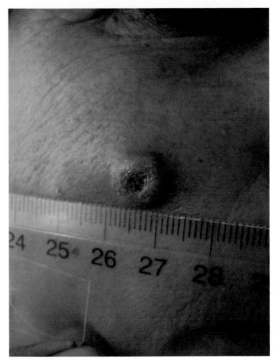

Figure 10.3.2 Keratoacanthoma on the right cheek. Quickly growing lesion, approximately 6 weeks. Examination is typical dome-shaped erythematous nodule with central keratin plug.

Aetiology/Pathology

Malignant melanomas result from both genetic and environmental factors:

- Genetic: Family history, fair skin type
- Environmental: Excessive UV radiation

Clinical presentation

Early skin melanomas are often asymptomatic and may not be noticed by the patient.

When taking a history, it is important to refer to the Glasgow 7-point checklist (see box) in order to differentiate the lesion from benign or atypical naevi.

Examination

Examination of the lesions should be conducted using the ABCDE criteria, which will help differentiate malignant from benign lesions (see box).

ABCDE Criteria

Asymmetry of lesion
Border (irregular)
Colour (variegated)
Diameter >6 mm
Enlargement/**E**volution

Glasgow 7-Point Checklist

Change in size (2 points)

Change in shape (2 points)

Change in colour (2 points)

Diameter >7 mm (1 point)

Inflammation 1 point)

Oozing (1 point)

Change in sensation (1 point)

Investigations

Dermatoscopy, histopathology and excision biopsy are used to diagnose a malignant melanoma. The excision biopsy (complete removal of the lesion with 2-mm clinical margin) is used to calculate the Breslow thickness (vertical diameter in mm from the granular cell layer to the deepest melanoma cell).

If the Breslow thickness is >1 mm, then additional investigations (FBC, LDH, LFTs, CXR, CT abdomen and pelvis, sentinel lymph node biopsy) are needed to detect potential metastases.

Management

If a patient scores 3 or above on the Glasgow seven-point checklist they should be referred down the suspected skin cancer referral pathway for an appointment within 2 weeks.

Malignant melanomas can be managed by wide local excision (treatment of choice). If there is metastatic disease, then chemotherapy and radiotherapy can be used.

REFERENCE

National Institute for Health and Care Excellence. NICE Guidelines Skin Cancer: Recognition and Referral. https://cks.nice.org.uk/skin-cancers-recognition-and-referral

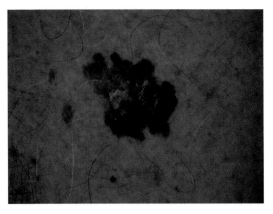

Figure 10.3.3 Superficial spreading malignant melanoma on the chest. Asymmetric flat lesion with irregular border (polycyclic), varying colours.

DERMATOLOGY: QUESTIONS

10.1 ECZEMA

1. Which surfaces does eczema typically affect?
2. What are the treatment options available for a flare of atopic eczema?
3. What are the complications of atopic eczema?

10.2 PSORIASIS

1. What are the nail changes that may be found in psoriasis?
2. Patients with psoriasis are at increased risk of which conditions?

3. What are the medical treatment options for the treatment of psoriasis as recommended by NICE?

10.3 SKIN CANCER

1. What is the main risk factor for the development of skin cancer?
2. What is the main differential diagnosis for a patient presenting with a squamous cell carcinoma?
3. What does the ABCDE criteria stand for in the assessment of pigmented lesions?
4. Is there any known precancerous condition leading to development of a BCC?

Orthopaedics

11.1 OSTEOARTHRITIS

DEFINITION

Osteoarthritis (OA) is a disorder characterised by the progressive loss of articular cartilage and remodelling of the underlying bone and formation of osteophytes, which most commonly affects the knees, hips and small joints of the hands.

EPIDEMIOLOGY

OA is the most common arthropathy and is a leading cause of pain and disability in the UK. The prevalence of OA of the knees, hips and hands increases with age. There is evidence that symptomatic knee OA occurs in 15% of adults over 55 years of age and there is a radiographic incidence of >80% in those over 75.

AETIOLOGY

OA has a multifactorial aetiology and can be primary (with no obvious cause) or secondary (to trauma, infiltrative disease or connective tissue diseases).

Risk factors include obesity, advancing age, trauma, female sex and occupation. In individuals predisposed to OA, repetitive joint motion is a risk.

PATHOLOGY

The pathogenesis of OA is more complicated than a wear-and-tear phenomenon but this is how patients (and doctors) often perceive it. Research suggests that chondrocytes in articular cartilage are activated by an unknown trigger and release enzymes that break down the cartilage and expose the underlying bone.

CLINICAL PRESENTATION

Patients report pain when using the affected joints that eases with rest. The affected joints may also become stiff with rest.

EXAMINATION

Perform a 'Look, Feel, Move' musculoskeletal examination of the affected joints.

Look: Nodes (Heberden's nodes on the distal interphalangeal joints [DIPs]), muscle wasting.

Feel: Joint effusion.

Move: Crepitus and reduced range of movement.

Always complete your musculoskeletal examination by mentioning that you would ideally examine the joint above and below the affected joint as well as completing a neurovascular examination.

INVESTIGATIONS

OA is a clinical diagnosis and can be made clinically if the patient is over 45 years of age. Investigations are primarily used to rule out other conditions (e.g. FBC [infection], ESR, bone profile [$\uparrow Ca^{2+}$], rheumatoid factor/anti-CCP).

X-rays of OA are common to see in finals. The x-ray changes associated with OA can be remembered by the mnemonic **LOSS: L**oss of joint space, **O**steophytes, **S**ubchondral cysts, **S**ubchondral sclerosis.

DIFFERENTIAL DIAGNOSIS

Table 11.1.1 presents the differential diagnosis for osteoarthritis.

MANAGEMENT

Chronic disease

Non-pharmacological

- Educate the patient about their condition and its progression
- Advise on joint protection and emphasise the importance of strengthening and aerobic exercise
- Weight loss for patients who are overweight
- Non-pharmacological interventions include:
  - Local heat and ice packs
  - Joint supports
  - Physiotherapy
  - Transcutaneous nerve stimulation

Pharmacological

- NICE advises working up a 'pain ladder' when providing analgesia for OA:
  - Paracetamol +/− topical NSAIDs/capsaicin (for hand or knee OA)
  - Addition of a weak opioid regularly
  - Use of a regular oral NSAID and a proton pump inhibitor
  - Use of intra-articular steroid injections

Table 11.1.1 Differential diagnosis for osteoarthritis

Hand OA	Hip OA	Knee OA
De Quervain's tenosynovitis	Trochanteric bursitis	All causes of hip pain (as can refer as knee pain)
Rheumatoid arthritis	Nerve entrapment (e.g. lumbar radiculopathy or lateral femoral cutaneous nerve)	Chondromalacia patellae
Gout	Lumbar spinal stenosis	Meniscal tear
	Iliotibial band syndrome	Ligament tear (such as ACL tear)

Surgical

- If the patient is fit for surgery and whose symptoms are not managed with medical treatment, consider referring patient for a surgical procedure.

- Two of the most common procedures that are asked about in finals are a total hip and total knee replacement. The complications of both are summarised in *Table 11.1.2*.

REFERENCE

National Institute for Health and Care Excellence. *NICE Guideline Osteoarthritis*. https://www.nice.org.uk/guidance/cg177

Table 11.1.2 Complications of joint replacement

Total hip replacement complications	Total knee replacement complications
Intraoperative: Acetabulum fracture	Intraoperative: Tibial fracture
Immediate: Dislocation	Immediate: Vascular injury
Early: DVT/infection/sciatic nerve palsy	Early: DVT/PE, Peroneal nerve palsy, infection
Late: Infection, compartment syndrome, leg-length discrepancy	Late: Infection, instability

11.2 HIP FRACTURE

DEFINITION

A hip fracture, or a fractured neck of femur (NOF), is a fracture of the proximal femur that extends to 5 cm below the lesser trochanter). It is the most common reason for admission to the orthopaedic trauma ward.

EPIDEMIOLOGY

Hip fractures are a major public health issue due to the ageing population. Approximately 75,000 hip fractures occur each year in the UK, causing a significant financial burden. They are much more common in the older population (average age 84 for men and 83 for women) and around 75% of fractures occur in women. Mortality is high for hip fractures, with one-third of patients dying within 12 months following the fracture.

AETIOLOGY

Hip fractures usually occur following trauma (which may be minor in patients with osteoporosis). Examples of trauma may include a fall onto the hip, direct blow to the hip or high-energy trauma (e.g. vehicle accident).

Other risk factors for sustaining a hip fracture include increasing age, osteoporosis (see Section 5.5), osteo-malacia and a history of falls (and risk factors for falls, e.g. poor vision, dementia etc.).

PATHOLOGY

Hip fractures are classically divided into whether they occur inside the femoral capsule (intracapsular) or outside the capsule (extracapsular). The femoral capsule is composed of three ligaments (iliofemoral, ischiofemoral and pubofemoral) that run from the acetabular margins proximally and insert onto the intertrochanteric line distally.

The main blood supply to the head of the femur comes from vessels that travel underneath the capsule along the femoral neck. This blood supply is mainly from the trochanteric anastomosis, which has contributions from the lateral and medial circumflex femoral arteries as well as the superior and inferior gluteal artery (Figure 11.2.1). If the hip fracture occurs within the femoral capsule (e.g. an intracapsular fracture), the blood supply to the head of the femur is often compromised, especially if it is a displaced fracture. If the blood supply to the head of the femur is compromised, avascular necrosis can occur.

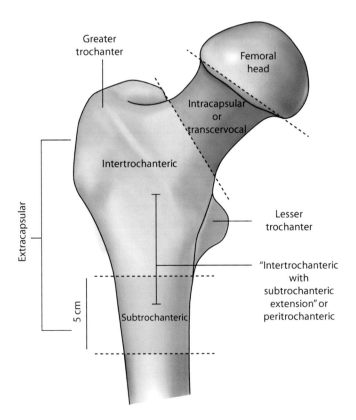

Figure 11.2.1 Anatomy of femoral neck.

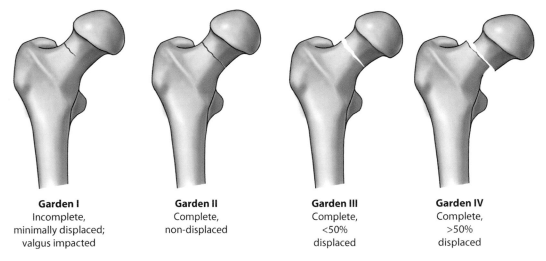

| **Garden I** | **Garden II** | **Garden III** | **Garden IV** |
| Incomplete, minimally displaced; valgus impacted | Complete, non-displaced | Complete, <50% displaced | Complete, >50% displaced |

Figure 11.2.2 Garden classification of intrascapular neck fractures.

Intracapsular fractures can be divided by the Garden classification (Figure 11.2.2):

- Garden I: Incomplete and nondisplaced fracture
- Garden II: Complete and nondisplaced fracture
- Garden III: Complete fracture with partial displacement
- Garden IV: Complete fracture with total displacement

CLINICAL PRESENTATION

Patients may present following a fall or trauma with pain in the hip or groin and limited ability to move the hip. If patients are immobile or arthritic, they may have trouble getting up off the ground following a fall and may be at risk of rhabdomyolysis.

EXAMINATION

The classic examination findings for a hip fracture are pain in the affected hip, inability to weight bear on the affected leg, limited range of hip movement and the affected leg being shortened and externally rotated.

INVESTIGATIONS

The diagnosis of a hip fracture is made from a hip x-ray. The majority of investigations that will be needed are presurgery bloods following a general systems examination.

- Bedside tests: Urinalysis (diabetes/UTI – hypoglycaemia/infection can cause falls in the elderly), ECG (arrhythmias).
- Bloods: FBC (check Hb and platelets), LFTs (check nutrition status/albumin), calcium (underlying malignancy), U&Es (to help guide anaesthetic choice and detect any AKI), clotting (as may affect time to heal), group and save (anticipatory blood matching for surgery), glucose (underlying diabetes).
- Imaging: CXR (detect any underlying pneumonia).

If a patient has been on the floor for a prolonged period of time and is at risk of rhabdomyolysis, check their CK level and their U&Es (rhabdomyolysis can cause ↑ K+ and an AKI which can also cause ↑ K+).

DIFFERENTIAL DIAGNOSIS

The differential diagnosis for hip fractures includes severe osteoarthritis, femoral shaft/pelvic fractures, septic arthritis, reactive arthritis, psoas abscess and radiculopathy.

MANAGEMENT

General fracture management can be remembered by the **4 Rs** (see box).

Surgical management is usually indicated for hip fractures (both intracapsular and extracapsular).

Once a hip fracture is suspected analgesia should be given. Options include paracetamol, opioids or nerve blocks (e.g. femoral nerve blocks) prior to surgery.

- Extracapsular fractures are not at risk of avascular necrosis and are usually treated with internal fixation with either an extramedullary plate or an intramedullary nail.
- Patients with a non-displaced intracapsular fracture and no comorbidities may also be treated with internal fixation. If patients do have major illness or advanced organ-specific disease, then a hemiarthroplasty is offered.
- Patients with a displaced intracapsular fracture are treated with either a total hip replacement or a hemiarthroplasty.
  - Patients should be offered a total hip replacement if they were able to walk independently prior to the fall, have no cognitive impairment and are medically fit for the procedure.

Following surgery, patients are managed using a multidisciplinary approach (e.g. orthogeriatrician, physiotherapist, occupational therapist) and are encouraged to mobilise the day following surgery with a physiotherapist.

Complications of fractures include tissue damage (haemorrhage, shock, infection, rhabdomyolysis), compartment syndrome (increase in pressure within a closed fascial compartment), neurological damage (e.g. neuropraxia, pain), malunion and avascular necrosis. (For specific hip surgery complications see Section 11.1.)

The 4 Rs of fracture management

Resuscitation: Using an ABCDE approach. Contaminant should be removed and any wounds dressed.

Reduction (if required): Some fractures can be reduced under anaesthetic using traction, manipulation or open reduction.

Restriction: Limb held in position to allow fracture to heal (e.g. use of plaster, slings, splints, nails).

Rehabilitation: Promotion of movement to reduce muscle loss and reduce risk of thrombosis.

ORTHOPAEDICS: QUESTIONS

OSTEOARTHRITIS

1. Name three features on examination that would be suggestive of hip osteoarthritis.

2. What are the x-ray features of an osteoarthritic joint?

3. What non-pharmacological therapies are available to treat osteoarthritis?

4. What pharmacological therapies are available to treat osteoarthritis?

5. What are the specific complications of a total knee replacement?

HIP FRACTURES

1. Name three risk factors for the having a hip fracture.

2. What types of hip fracture are there?

3. What is the Garden classification?

4. Which investigations should be performed in a patient prior to hip fracture surgery?

5. Name three complications of fractures.

CHAPTER **12**

General Surgery

12.1 GALLSTONES

DEFINITION

Gallstones are solid deposits that form from bile within the gallbladder.

EPIDEMIOLOGY

Gallstones are common in Western countries, with prevalence rates reported between 5%–30%. Risk factors for developing gallstones include obesity, female gender, increasing age, hypertriglyceridaemia, diabetes, HRT, smoking and Crohn's disease. It is estimated that 8% of adults over the age of 40 have gallstones.

AETIOLOGY/PATHOLOGY

Bile contains cholesterol, pigments (from Hb) and phospholipids. A change in the concentration of any of these constituents can lead to the formation of different stones. Cholesterol stones are the most common type and are large, whereas pigment stones are rare and smaller. A mixed stone picture can also occur.

CLINICAL PRESENTATION

Most people with gallstones (90%) are asymptomatic. Of these people, 4% develop symptoms each year.

Gallstones can present in a number of ways:

Biliary colic: Contraction of the gallbladder against a stone in the neck of the gallbladder causing RUQ and epigastric pain that is continuous (unlike other types of colic). Classically caused by eating a fatty meal (which releases CCK from the duodenum that causes the gallbladder to contract).

Acute cholecystitis: Inflammation around an obstructed gallstone. As for biliary colic + pyrexia, tachycardia and tachypnoea. Murphy's sign may be positive (see later). May have secondary bacterial infection.

Ascending cholangitis: Infection in the biliary tract from obstructed gallstones that clinically manifests as **Charcot's triad** (pain + jaundice + rigors).

Mucocele: Neck of the gallbladder obstructed by a stone that becomes impacted, which leads to distension of the gallbladder. May be asymptomatic or present as a RUQ mass if it becomes infected.

Acute pancreatitis: See Section 12.2.

Gallstone ileus: Small bowel obstruction secondary to gallstones which have entered the bowel via a fistula. The narrowest part of the small bowel is the ileocaecal valve, which is where stones may impact.

EXAMINATION

Patients may have a number of signs on examination depending on the presentation of their gallstones.

General inspection:

- Jaundice (acute cholecystitis, ascending cholangitis)
- Distended abdomen (small bowel obstruction secondary to a gallstone ileus)
- Peritonitic (shallow breathing, prefer to be lying down)

Palpation:

- Tenderness on palpation of the right upper quadrant/epigastric region
- Murphy's sign positive:
  - To elicit Murphy's sign place two fingers over the RUQ and ask the patient to breath in. This will cause pain in the RUQ and arrest of inspiration as the gallbladder moves inferiorly towards your hand. The test is only said to be positive if the same test in the LUQ does not cause pain

INVESTIGATIONS

Bedside: ECG (ACS can present with epigastric pain and shares similar risk factors to gallstone disease).

Bloods: FBC (↑ WCC), LFTs (↑ ALP), ↑ GGT (obstructed picture), ↑ bilirubin (if cholecystitis/cholangitis).

Imaging: USS abdomen, AXR (10% of gallstones are radio-opaque), CXR (exclude other pathology [e.g. right basal pneumonia] and pneumoperitoneum).

Invasive: MRCP (used to find stones, whereas ERCP is used to remove them).

DIFFERENTIAL DIAGNOSIS

The differential diagnosis for gallstones disease includes, but is not limited to, peptic ulcer disease, gastritis, GORD, pancreatitis (from other causes), hepatitis, gallbladder cancer, pancreatic cancer, gastrointestinal cancer.

MANAGEMENT

Management will depend on the presentation of gallstones.

For biliary colic, avoid triggers (e.g. dietary changes) and analgesia (NICE recommend diclofenac IM unless contraindicated), which may be followed by elective cholecystectomy.

Patients with symptomatic gallstone disease will usually be admitted to secondary care to undergo a cholecystectomy ± IV antibiotics if there is evidence of bacterial infection (e.g. ascending cholangitis).

A cholecystectomy is a common procedure for patients to undertake so it is important to know about for finals. They can be performed either via an open procedure (using a Kocher incision) or laparoscopically (Figure 12.1.1). During the procedure, the operating surgeon will first identify the cystic artery, which sits within Calot's triangle (formed by the lower liver border, the cystic duct and the common hepatic duct). The cystic artery is ligated, and the gallbladder is then dissected.

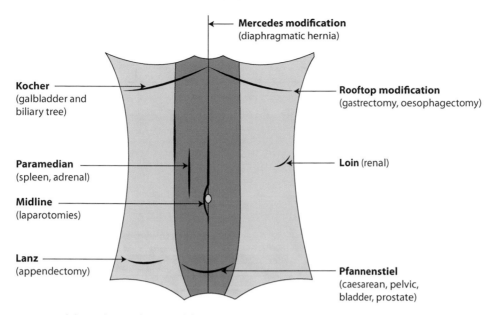

Mercedes modification
(diaphragmatic hernia)

Kocher
(galbladder and
biliary tree)

Rooftop modification
(gastrectomy, oesophagectomy)

Paramedian
(spleen, adrenal)

Loin (renal)

Midline
(laparotomies)

Lanz
(appendectomy)

Pfannenstiel
(caesarean, pelvic,
bladder, prostate)

Figure 12.1.1 Abdominal surgical scars and their indications.

Specific complications of a cholecystectomy include:

- Bleeding from the cystic or hepatic artery
- Bile leakage
- Bile duct injury
- Damage to the intestine
- Postcholecystectomy syndrome (abdominal pain, dyspepsia, diarrhoea), which is thought to be secondary to retained small gallstones or sphincter of Oddi dysfunction

12.2 PANCREATITIS

DEFINITION

Pancreatitis is an inflammatory process of the pancreas that may involve other local organ systems and retro-peritoneal tissue. It can occur acutely or chronically.

EPIDEMIOLOGY

Acute pancreatitis has an estimated incidence of 150–420/1,000,000 in the UK, which appears to be rising.

AETIOLOGY

The causes of pancreatitis can be remembered by the well-known mnemonic, **GET SMASH³ED**: **G**allstones (most common cause in women), **E**thanol (most common cause in men), **T**rauma, **S**teroids, **M**umps (other viruses include Coxsackie B/Epstein–Barr), **A**utoimmune (e.g. polyarteritis nodosa/SLE), **S**corpion venom and snake bites, **H**ypertriglyceridaemia, **H**ypercalcaemia, **H**ypothermia, **E**RCP, **D**rugs (azathioprine, bendroflumethiazide, furosemide, steroids, sodium valproate).

PATHOLOGY

The pathogenesis of pancreatitis involves the abnormal activation of digestive enzymes within the pancreas. Pancreatic enzymes are usually secreted into the small bowel as proenzymes before being cleaved into their active form (e.g. trypsinogen being cleaved to trypsin). In pancreatitis, these enzymes become active within the pancreas and lead to inflammation, oedema and cell death. The fluid shifts caused by the inflammatory response cause hypovolaemia as extracellular fluid is moved to the gut and to the 'third space' e.g. peritoneal cavity and retroperitoneal space.

CLINICAL PRESENTATION

Acute pancreatitis classically presents with vomiting and epigastric/central abdominal pain that radiates to the back (the pancreas is retroperitoneal), which may be relieved by sitting forwards. There may be a history of a cause of the pancreatitis (e.g. established gallstone disease, recent ERCP procedure).

EXAMINATION

Signs on examination of patients with acute pancreatitis can vary widely. Due to the third space fluid loss, patients may present in shock ($\uparrow$ HR, $\downarrow$ BP) and may be peritonitic on examination. Abdominal distension may be observed due to the leakage of fluid into the retroperitoneum causing the abdominal contents to be pushed forward.

The eponymous signs associated with pancreatitis are Cullen's sign (periumbilical bruising) and Grey–Turner's sign (flank bruising). These are caused by blood vessel autodigestion and retroperitoneal haemorrhage.

INVESTIGATIONS

Bedside: ECG (to investigate for ACS).

Bloods: FBC ($\uparrow$ WCC), serum amylase/lipase ($\uparrow\uparrow$), ABG (monitor oxygenation and acid–base), LFTs (may be $\uparrow$ in gallstone/hepatic disease), bone profile ($\uparrow$ Ca^{2+} is a cause of pancreatitis), lipids ($\uparrow$ triglycerides), autoimmune screen (if autoimmune cause suspected), U&Es and blood glucose are needed to predict severity (see later).

Imaging: AXR (lack of psoas shadow indicates $\uparrow$ retroperitoneal fluid), CXR (rule out perforation), USS abdomen (look for evidence of gallstones); CT is used to assess severity.

Invasive: ERCP (potentially if gallstones suspected).

DIFFERENTIAL DIAGNOSIS

The differential diagnosis of acute pancreatitis includes biliary colic, acute cholecystitis, ascending cholangitis, viral hepatitis, gastroenteritis, perforated peptic ulcer, bowel obstruction, ischaemic bowel, ruptured abdominal aortic aneurysm or myocardial infarction.

MANAGEMENT

Patients need to be managed with an ABCDE approach.

Intravenous access is gained to give plentiful fluids to counter third-space losses. Patients are made nil by mouth and may be given an NG tube (to decrease pancreatic stimulation).

Analgesics are given and antibiotics if there is associated cholangitis or acute infection.

If there is an underlying cause identified (e.g. gallstones), then an urgent therapeutic ERCP can be organised.

There are a number of scores used to predict the severity of pancreatitis. The modified Glasgow criteria is frequently used and can be remembered by the mnemonic **PANCREAS**:

P$_a$O2	<8 kPa
Age	>55
Neutrophils	>15 × 109
Calcium	<2 mmol/L
Raised urea	>16 mmol/L
Enzymes (LDH)	>600 IU/L
Albumin	<32 g/L
Sugars	>10 mmol/L

A score of more than three detected within 48 hours of onset suggests severe pancreatitis and transfer to a high-dependency/intensive care unit.

Other pancreatitis severity scores include the Ranson criteria and the APACHE score.

The Ranson score looks at clinical parameters on admission (age, white cells, glucose, AST, LDH) and parameters 48 hours later (calcium, haematocrit, oxygen, blood urea nitrogen, base excess and fluids).

The APACHE score looks at clinical parameters (haemorrhagic peritoneal fluid, obesity, organ failure, shock, hypoxia, oliguria, calcium or albumin) to make a prediction of mortality.

Complications

The complications of pancreatitis can be divided into early and late.

Early complications: Shock and renal failure, acute respiratory distress syndrome, hypocalcaemia, hyperglycaemia.

Late complications: **Pancreatic pseudocyst** (fluid in the lesser sac – patients present weeks later with pyrexia, an abdominal mass and persistently raised amylase). **Pancreatic necrosis** (due to loss of blood supply to the pancreas causes necrosis and subsequent infection). **Type 1 diabetes mellitus** (due to an absolute insulin deficiency from beta cell destruction). **Chronic pancreatitis** (recurrent attacks of pancreatitis that requires pancreatic enzyme supplementation).

12.3 HERNIAS AND GROIN LUMPS

DEFINITION

A hernia is defined as the protrusion of a viscus, or part of a viscus, through the walls of its containing cavity into an abnormal position. Examples of hernias include groin hernias (inguinal and femoral), epigastric, paraumbilical, incisional and spigelian (which occur through the *linea semilumaris* of the rectus sheath).

EPIDEMIOLOGY

The most common types of hernia are groin hernias (75%), the most common of which are inguinal hernias in both men and women. Femoral hernias are more common in women. Inguinal hernias can be further subdivided into direct (less common – 20%) and indirect (more common – 80%) inguinal hernias.

The risk factors for developing a hernia include chronic raised intraabdominal pressure (e.g. chronic cough, constipation, straining), obesity, age, severe muscular effort (e.g. heavy lifting) and previous abdominal surgery.

AETIOLOGY/PATHOLOGY

Inguinal hernias are classified by where in the inguinal canal they emerge and their position relative to the inferior epigastric vessels (which branch from the external iliac) in Hesselbach's triangle. Knowledge of the relevant anatomy is crucial for differentiating between inguinal and femoral hernias (Figures 12.3.1, 12.3.2).

Indirect inguinal hernias emerge through the **deep inguinal ring** along with the structures of the spermatic cord and are as a result **lateral to the inferior epigastric vessels**. Some indirect inguinal hernias occur due to a patent processus vaginalis, which usually obliterates in childhood. The deep inguinal ring can be found at the **midpoint of the inguinal ligament** (1 cm above and lateral to the femoral pulse at the mid-inguinal point).

Direct inguinal hernias enter the inguinal canal through a weakness or defect in its posterior wall more medially and as a result emerge medially to the inferior epigastric vessels within Hesselbach's triangle.

Femoral hernias emerge through the femoral canal medially to the femoral vessels. Because of the position of the femoral canal, femoral hernias can be differentiated from inguinal hernias by the **position of the pubic tubercle**. Femoral hernias emerge **below and lateral to the pubic tubercle**, while inguinal hernias occur **above and medial** to the pubic tubercle.

As these hernias are the protrusion through the abdominal cavity, they contain bowel and blood supply. If the bowel within the hernia becomes obstructed, this can lead to a presentation of bowel obstruction. If the blood supply within the hernia is compromised, then the hernia may become strangulated. Due to the narrow nature of the femoral canal because of the lacunar ligament, femoral hernias are more likely to strangulate than inguinal hernias.

CLINICAL PRESENTATION

Groin hernias typically present as a lump in the groin that classically appears on straining/lifting and disappears on lying down or when pressed. There may be pain in the groin due to the pressure from the hernia or due to a complication (obstruction or strangulation).

EXAMINATION

To examine for a groin lump, ask the patient to lie down and expose their abdomen, groins and legs.

Inspect for the lump and for scars from previous surgery.

Examine the external genitalia and both groins to ascertain whether this is a groin lump or a scrotal lump.

If there is a scrotal swelling which **you cannot get above**, this may be due to an **inguinoscrotal hernia** (an indirect hernia that has extended to the scrotum). If you can get above it, it may be a cord or testicular lump.

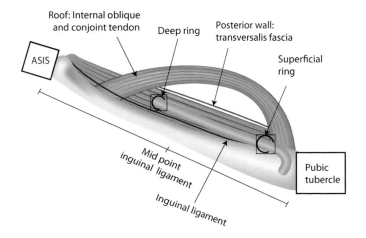

Figure 12.3.1 Anatomy of inguinal canal.

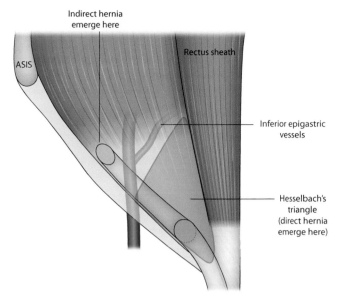

Figure 12.3.2   Hesselbach's triangle.

Hernia examination

Hernias exhibit four features: (1) cannot get above them, (2) cough impulse, (3) reducible and (4) bowel sounds.

Find your two key landmarks, the **pubic tubercle** and the **deep inguinal ring** at the midpoint of the inguinal ligament.

Palpate and comment on the features of the hernia.

Ask the patient to cough and feel for the presence of a cough impulse (hernia will expand).

Auscultate the hernia for bowel sounds.

Ask the patient to reduce the hernia (if possible) and identify the **pubic tubercle**. Once reduced, ask the patient to cough. Ascertain whether the lump appears **above and medial to the pubic tubercle** (inguinal hernia) or **below and lateral** (femoral hernia). Repeat the examination with the patient standing.

If you think there is an inguinal hernia or if you are asked to differentiate between direct and indirect, **reduce the hernia** and **occlude the deep inguinal ring** at the midpoint of the inguinal ligament. Ask the patient to either **cough** or **stand** – if the hernia **reappears despite occlusion of the deep inguinal ring**, this indicates that the hernia is **direct**. If the hernia **does not reappear and is contained**, this indicates that the hernia is **indirect**.

The only true way to ascertain between an indirect and direct inguinal hernia is during **surgery**.

INVESTIGATIONS

The major investigation for differentiating between the causes of a groin lump is a USS. Indications for an urgent USS scan of the groin and tests include a hydrocele detected in a man 20–34 years of age (highest risk for testicular cancer), body of testis cannot be distinguished, cannot distinguish whether swelling is testicular or extra-testicular, persistent testicular symptoms, history of trauma/scrotal pain or diagnostic uncertainty. If you suspect a sinister cause for a groin lump (e.g. widespread lymphadenopathy in haematological malignancy or hard testis in testicular cancer), then bloods should be taken looking at white blood counts or testicular cancer tumour markers (B-hCG, AFP, LDH).

DIFFERENTIAL DIAGNOSIS

The differential diagnosis for a groin lump includes groin hernia, lymphadenopathy, testicular cancer, testicular torsion (or torsion of appendix testis or appendix epididymis), epididymo-orchitis, varicocele, hydrocele, haematocele and an epididymal cyst.

MANAGEMENT

If a patient presents with evidence of strangulation (e.g. pain out of proportion to clinical features, irreducible hernia) or obstruction, this requires urgent surgical exploration and repair.

The majority of inguinal hernias are managed surgically with either an open or laparoscopic repair to either excise the sac (herniotomy) to reduce the hernia and repair the posterior wall and deep inguinal ring (herniorrhaphy) usually with the insertion of a nylon mesh. Patients are advised to lose weight (if overweight) and stop smoking prior to the operation and warned that the inguinal hernia may reoccur.

Specific complications of surgery include damage to local structures (e.g. ilioinguinal nerve → pain/paraesthesia, damage to the blood supply to the testicle or damage to the vas deferens).

Femoral hernias are almost always surgically managed due to their high risk of strangulation. The procedure involves reduction of the hernia and surgical narrowing of the femoral ring using sutures. Specific complications of surgery include damage to the femoral vessels (the vein is nearest the hernia) and the femoral nerve.

12.4 BREAST CANCER

DEFINITION
Breast cancer is a malignant neoplasm arising from breast tissue.

EPIDEMIOLOGY
Breast cancer is now the most common cancer in the UK, with approximately 50,000 new cases diagnosed every year.

AETIOLOGY
Breast cancer has a multifactorial aetiology with a strong familial component. Approximately 10% of breast cancers are familial (increased risk with first-degree relative who has developed breast cancer) and approximately one-half of these are associated with the BRCA1 (17q) and BRCA2 (13q) mutations.

There are a number of environmental risk factors for developing breast cancer, which include oestrogen exposure (see box), previous breast cancer, increasing age and not breast feeding.

> ### Factors ↑ oestrogen exposure
> - Nulliparity
> - First pregnancy >30 years
> - Early menarche
> - Late menopause
> - Hormone replacement therapy
> - COCP pill use
> - Obesity

PATHOLOGY
Breast cancers are predominantly adenocarcinomas, which can be further subdivided into ductal (85%) or lobular (15%). Breast cancers may originate as either **ductal carcinoma in situ (DCIS)** or **lobular carcinoma in situ (LCIS)**, which are non-invasive premalignant conditions.

The most common type of breast cancer is invasive ductal carcinoma followed by invasive lobular carcinoma.

Other types of breast cancer involve medullary (younger patients, BRCA1 association), colloid/mucinous (older patients) and inflammatory (rapidly progressive, erythematous and oedematous).

CLINICAL PRESENTATION
Breast cancers are usually identified either through screening (see box) or in patients presenting with a breast lump (see box for NICE referral guidelines). Other presenting features include breast pain (usually with lump), nipple skin changes (red eczema-like changes on and around the nipple suggest Paget's disease of the breast), nipple discharge or with symptoms of metastases (e.g. bone pain).

> ### Breast screening
> - Women 47–73 years old offered mammography every 3 years
> - High-risk women offered earlier screening
> - If abnormal, women recalled for triple assessment

EXAMINATION
Always ask for a chaperone for intimate examinations.

Inspection: Observe for any asymmetry between the breasts and any overlying skin changes, which may include inflammation, ulceration, skin retraction or peau d'orange (orange peel skin – occurs due to lymphatic obstruction resulting in oedema and dimples from hair follicles in the breast). Observe for any nipple changes (flaking, deviation, inversion, discharge).

Manoeuvres can be used to accentuate any masses: (1) ask the patient to raise their arms above their head (skin tethering becomes more apparent), and (2) press their hands against their hips (tenses pectoral muscles to accentuate tethering to the chest wall).

Palpation: Examine the asymptomatic breast first with the patient lying at a 45-degree angle. Using the flat surface of three fingers, examine the breast using a systematic approach (using either the clock face method – examining each 'hour' of the breast, or the spiral method – starting at the nipple and working outwards in a circular motion). Palpate the axillary tail (of Spence) and the axilla and supraclavicular fossa for any lymphadenopathy.

If you find a lump, it is important to know how to describe it:

- State its position (e.g. upper outer quadrant)
- Size (e.g. 2 cm × 4 cm)
- Shape (e.g. spherical, irregular/regular)
- Consistency (e.g. smooth, firm)
- Overlying skin (e.g. erythema, ulceration)
- Mobility (e.g. freely mobile or fixed)
- Transillumination (e.g. indicating fluid contents)

> ### NICE Referral Guidelines for Breast Cancer (https://cks.nice.org.uk/breast-cancer-recognition-and-referral)
>
> Consider a 2-week wait referral if a patient is:
> - ≥30 with unexplained breast lump
> - ≥50 with unilateral nipple changes (e.g. discharge, retraction)

INVESTIGATIONS

The investigations for a breast lump typically undergo a 'triple assessment', which involves:

- Clinical examination
- Imaging: USS (if <35) or mammography (if >35)
- Pathological analysis: Fine-needle aspiration or tissue biopsy

If a breast cancer is identified, additional tests for hormone receptor status (oestrogen/progesterone) and HER2 receptor status are performed, as receptor positive cancers can be given adjuvant therapy (see box).

The tumour marker that may be raised in breast cancer is CA15-3.

DIFFERENTIAL DIAGNOSIS

The differential diagnosis for a breast lump can be found in *Table 12.4.1*.

STAGING

Breast cancer staging helps guide management and is split into four separate stages:

- Stage 1: Confined to breast; mobile; no lymph nodes
- Stage 2: Stage 1 + nodes in ipsilateral axilla
- Stage 3: Stage 2 + fixation to muscle (not chest wall); LNs fixed

Table 12.4.1 Differential diagnosis of a breast lump

Condition	Features
Fibroadenoma	Young patients (20s–30s) Painless smooth breast lump, freely mobile (also known as breast mice)
Fat necrosis	Breast lump occurring following a fall; more common in overweight patients
Duct ectasia	Classically a smoker who presents with thick white/green nipple discharge
Mastitis	Painful, red breast that classically occurs in breastfeeding women
Breast abscess	Painful, erythematous, swollen lump in the breast with fever
Paget's disease of the nipple	Unilateral erythematous scaly skin changes over the nipple; breast lump may be found underlying

- Stage 4: Complete fixation to chest wall and metastases
  - Breast cancer most commonly spreads to the bones, lungs, liver and brain.

MANAGEMENT

A number of options can be offered to patients depending on their staging and receptor status.

Carcinomas in situ (e.g. DCIS/LCIS) are usually treated with breast-conserving surgery.

Stage 1 and 2 cancers are usually offered surgery with adjuvant therapy (see box).

- Surgery can either be a mastectomy or a wide local excision (WLE)
- Factors that may guide choice include the type and size of tumour (e.g. large or multifocal lesions → mastectomy, whereas small or solitary lesion → WLE)
- Patients treated with WLE are usually offered radiotherapy
- During surgery a sentinel node biopsy is performed (looking for lymph node involvement); if it is positive, axillary clearance or radiotherapy is performed
- Complications of surgery include lymphoedema, frozen shoulder and long thoracic nerve palsy

Stage 3 and 4 cancers are usually treated with chemotherapy or palliation with adjuvant therapy.

Adjuvant therapy

Hormone receptor positive

- If premenopausal, a selective oestrogen receptor modulator (e.g. tamoxifen) is offered
- If postmenopausal, an aromatase inhibitor (e.g. anastrozole) is offered
- **Note**: Tamoxifen ↑ risk of endometrial cancer and DVT; aromatase inhibitors ↑ risk of osteoporosis

HER2 positive

- Transtuzimab (Herceptin) is offered to patients who are HER2 positive
- **Note**: Transtuzimab is contraindicated in patients with heart disorders

12.5 COLORECTAL CARCINOMA

DEFINITION
Colorectal carcinoma is a malignant neoplasm of the large intestine.

EPIDEMIOLOGY
Colorectal carcinoma is the most common gastrointestinal cancer, the second most common cause of cancer deaths in the UK and the third most common cause of cancer overall. There are around 40,000 new colorectal cancers diagnosed every year in the UK; 45% are found in the rectum followed by 25% in the sigmoid colon.

AETIOLOGY
There are a number of predisposing factors for the development of colorectal carcinoma, which include neoplastic polyps (neoplastic proliferations with malignant potential), inflammatory bowel disease (UC>CD), low-fibre diet, smoking, previous cancer and familial cancer syndromes (familial adenomatous polyposis [FAP] and hereditary non-polyposis colorectal carcinoma [HNPCC] – both autosomal dominant).

PATHOLOGY
The majority of colorectal cancers are adenocarcinomas (95%) that originate from the epithelial cells of the large bowel due to a result of mutations in the Wnt signalling pathway. The most common mutated gene is the APC gene, and mutations in both APC genes leads to adenoma formation, which undergoes malignant transformation following further genetic mutations (e.g. in p53). Colorectal carcinomas can spread locally, by the lymphatic system, haematogenously (most commonly to liver, lung and bone) or transcolemically.

CLINICAL PRESENTATION
The clinical presentation of colorectal carcinoma largely depends on the location of the cancer.

Right-sided tumours: Present with weight loss and iron deficiency anaemia.

Left-sided tumours: Present with PR bleeding, altered bowel habit, tenesmus or large bowel obstruction.

Other symptoms suggestive of colorectal carcinoma include appetite loss, DVT, fatigue (due to anaemia) and abdominal pain (see box).

Two-week wait referral guidelines for colorectal cancer
- Iron deficiency anaemia ≥60
- Unexplained change in bowel habit ≥60
- Unexplained rectal bleeding ≥50
- Abdominal pain + weight loss ≥40

EXAMINATION
General examination may show **signs of iron deficiency anaemia** (pallor, koilonychias, angular stomatitis).

Palpation may reveal hepatomegaly (metastases). PR examination may reveal a **palpable mass**.

If you are examining a patient in a long case who has previously had an operation for colorectal cancer, you may be asked to examine the stoma, or comment on the type of surgery performed.

INVESTIGATIONS
Bedside: Fecal occult blood test.

Bloods: FBC (microcytic anaemia), LFTs (metastases), CEA (tumour marker).

Imaging: CXR (metastases), USS liver (metastases), CT/MRI (staging).

Invasive: Colonoscopy (visualise lesion and biopsy).

STAGING
There are two staging systems for colorectal carcinoma: the TNM (tumour, node, metastases) staging system and Dukes' classification.

TNM
- T1 Tumour confined to submucosa
- T2 Tumour grown into muscularis propria
- T3 Tumour grown into serosa
- T4 Tumour penetrated through serosa and peritoneal surface
- N0 No lymph node involvement
- N1 Up to three regional lymph nodes involved
- N2 Four or more regional lymph nodes involved
- M0 No metastases
- M1 Metastasis to distant organs

Dukes' classification
A. Tumour confined beneath muscularis mucosae (90% 5-year survival)
B. Tumour extension through muscularis mucosae (65% 5-year survival)
C. Involvement of regional lymph nodes (30% 5-year survival)
D. Distant metastases (<10% 5-year survival)

MANAGEMENT
The primary treatment of colorectal carcinoma is **surgery** and **resection** of the tumour. Adjunctive treatment options include radiotherapy and chemotherapy agents (e.g. capecitabine, oxaliplatin with 5-flurouracil).

The site and staging of the tumour dictate the surgical options used. The different procedures include:

- Right hemicolectomy for caecal, ascending and proximal transverse colon tumours
- Left hemicolectomy for distal transverse colon or descending colon tumours
- Sigmoid colectomy for sigmoid tumours
- Anterior resection for low sigmoid or high rectal tumours. If primary anastomosis cannot be made → **loop ileostomy** can be created while the bowel recovers before reattaching the bowel
- Total mesorectal excision for rectal tumours, with removal of surrounding fatty tissue and nodes (↑ survival)
- Abdominoperineal (AP) resection for low rectal tumours (≤8 cm from the anus). Results in an **end colostomy**
- Hartmann's procedure for patients presenting as an emergency with large bowel obstruction. Results in a temporary **end colostomy**. It is temporary and the two parts of the bowel are rejoined in a later surgery

Specific complications of surgery include damage to local vascular structures (bleeding) and damage to local nerves (e.g. risk of erectile dysfunction/vaginal lubrication in rectal surgery).

Stomas

A stoma is a surgically created opening in the body between the skin and a hollow viscus. There are three types (*Table 12.5.1*). Loop colostomies (or ileostomies) have two holes (as opposed to one) and are used to allow bowel to heal to allow the option of a future anastomosis.

When examining a stoma, note the **site** (RIF/LIF), the number of **openings** (loop [2] or end [1]), its **contents** (liquid/solid faeces or urine), and whether it has a **spout** or is **flush** with the skin. Perform an abdominal examination and at the site of the stoma and ask the patient to cough, looking for evidence of **herniation**.

Complications of a stoma include **high output** (dehydration and electrolyte disturbance e.g. ↓ K+), bowel obstruction, parastomal hernia, odour, skin irritation and psychological complications.

Patients need to alter their diet when they have a stoma (↑ fluids, ↓ fibre) and have a stoma nurse involved.

Bowel obstruction

Bowel obstruction can occur in the small or large bowel (*Table 12.5.2*). It is more common in the small bowel (80%).

The four cardinal features of bowel obstruction are vomiting, colic, absolute constipation and distension.

Other causes of lower GI bleeding

- Diverticular disease: Outpouchings of the large bowel usually secondary to a low-fibre diet. May become inflamed and infected leading to diverticulitis → can present with haemorrhage, peritonitis or perforation.
- Anorectal conditions (e.g. haemorrhoids, anal fissure).
- Angiodysplasia: Submucosal arteriovenous malformations that predominantly occur in the right colon.
- Colitis (e.g. ulcerative – see Section 3.2), ischaemia (compromised blood flow to bowel → ulceration and haemorrhage) or infective (e.g. *Campylobacter*).

Table 12.5.1 Different types of stomas

	Ileostomy	Colostomy	Urostomy
Location	RIF	LIF	RIF
Content	Liquid faeces	Solid faeces	Urine
Opening	Spout	Flush with skin	Flush with skin
Used in	Postcolectomy (**END**) (ulcerative colitis, FAP) Anterior resection (**LOOP**)	AP resection (**END**) Hartmann's procedure (**END**)	Cystectomy for bladder cancer

Table 12.5.2 Comparison of small vs. large bowel obstruction

Small bowel obstruction	Large bowel obstruction
Usually due to adhesions	Usually due to colorectal carcinoma or diverticulitis
Vomiting occurs early and there is ↑ pain	↑ Abdominal distension
AXR shows dilated small bowel proximal to the obstruction with *valvulae conniventes* (appear like stacked coins) CT is more sensitive than AXR	AXR shows colonic distension CT confirms the diagnosis
Treatment is conservative with IV fluids and NG tube (drip and suck)	Large bowel obstruction requires surgery and may result in a Hartmann's procedure

GENERAL SURGERY: QUESTIONS

12.1 GALLSTONES

1. What is the most common type of gallstones?
2. Name three ways in which gallstones can present.
3. What are the complications of a cholecystectomy?

12.2 PANCREATITIS

1. What are the causes of pancreatitis?
2. What scoring systems can be used to grade the severity of acute pancreatitis?
3. What are the complications of pancreatitis?

12.3 HERNIAS AND GROIN LUMPS

1. What is the difference aetiologically between indirect and direct inguinal hernias?
2. What are the borders and significance of Hesselbach's triangle?

3. What are the complications of inguinal hernia repair surgery?

12.4 BREAST CANCER

1. Name three risk factors for developing breast cancer.
2. What is involved in a triple assessment in a patient with a breast lump?
3. What are the treatment options for a patient with breast cancer?

12.5 COLORECTAL CANCER

1. How do right-sided and left-sided colorectal carcinomas classically present?
2. What are the risk factors for the development of colorectal carcinoma?
3. What are the complications of a stoma?

Urology

13.1 RENAL/URETERIC STONES

DEFINITION
Renal stones are the formation of stones in one or both of the kidneys, which may then pass down the ureters into the bladder. The term renal or ureteric colic is used to describe the pain caused by the obstruction of a ureter due to a renal stone.

EPIDEMIOLOGY
Renal stones are common, with 1 in 11 people (9%) getting stone symptoms during their lifetime. Men are slightly more often affected than women. They can occur at any age but the peak age for a first stone is around the age of 45 years.

AETIOLOGY
Renal stones occur when certain chemicals crystallise in the urine. This tends to occur when there is an excess of certain chemicals that are too concentrated due to a low volume of urine. The most common type are calcium-based stones (60%–80%) and are usually made up of a mixture of calcium oxalate and calcium phosphate. Other stone types include struvite (infection or triple-phosphate stones) (10%–15%), uric acid (5%–10%), cystine (1%) or others such as stones formed from certain drugs (e.g. indinavir/triamterene) (Table 13.1.1).

Risk factors for developing renal stones include family history, diet (especially if high in animal protein, salt and refined sugar), anatomically abnormal kidneys (e.g. horseshoe kidney), metabolic disease ($\uparrow$ Ca^{2+}, gout, cystinuria, renal tubular acidosis), metabolic syndrome (insulin resistance causes urine acidification), dehydration and chronic infection.

PATHOLOGY
Renal stones usually obstruct at one of three sites in the urinary tract (Figure 13.1.1):

- The pelvi-ureteric junction (PUJ)
- The mid-ureter where the ureter crosses the iliac vessels
- The vesico-ureteric junction (VUJ)

The obstruction in the ureter causes colic pain as peristaltic waves move down the ureters. The obstruction leads to prostaglandin secretion (causing vasodilation $\rightarrow$ diuresis $\rightarrow$ $\uparrow$ pressure in the kidney) and smooth muscle spasm of the ureter.

CLINICAL PRESENTATION
Patients usually present with renal colic $\pm$ nausea and vomiting. Renal colic is described as 'loin to groin' pain (in the direction of ureteric peristalsis) that comes and goes with waves of increasing severity. It usually starts as flank pain and slowly progresses towards the abdomen as the stone moves inferiorly. The pain can be referred to the testis in men and labia majora in women. Patients may also present with features of a UTI, haematuria (although renal stones will usually show blood on urinalysis) or urinary retention.

EXAMINATION
Patients may not be able to sit still with the pain (in contrast to peritonitis) and may be pale and sweaty. There may be tenderness on palpation of the abdomen.

INVESTIGATIONS
Bedside: Urinalysis (for blood/pH/nitrites/white cells).

Bloods: FBC (infection), U&Es (renal failure), bone profile (Ca^{2+}/PO$_4$$^{3-}$), uric acid and C-reactive protein.

Imaging: The investigation of choice is a non-contrast enhanced CT (CT-KUB).

DIFFERENTIAL DIAGNOSIS
The differential diagnosis for renal stones includes ruptured AAA, pyelonephritis, cholecystitis, pancreatitis, appendicitis, diverticulitis, bowel obstruction and testicular torsion.

MANAGEMENT
Immediate management for patients with renal stones is to provide adequate analgesia $\pm$ antiemetic. This is best achieved with non-steroidal anti-inflammatory drugs (NSAIDs), such as diclofenac IM, PR or orally, along with IV paracetamol. If there is evidence of

Table 13.1.1 Types of renal stones

Stone	Cause	Urine acidity	X-ray appearance
Calcium oxalate	$\uparrow$ Ca^{2+} in the urine (renal failure, nephrocalcinosis) or systemically (see Section 7.5 for hypercalcaemia)	Alkaline	Radio-opaque
Calcium phosphate	Metabolic causes (e.g. renal tubular acidosis [1 + 3])	Alkaline	Radio-opaque
Struvite	Urease-producing bacteria (associated with chronic infections – classically *Proteus* – causing staghorn calculi)	Alkaline	Slightly radio-opaque
Uric acid	Hyperuricaemia (see Section 5.4 for gout)	Acidic	Radiolucent
Cystine	Inherited renal tubular defect (cystinuria)	Normal	Radiodense

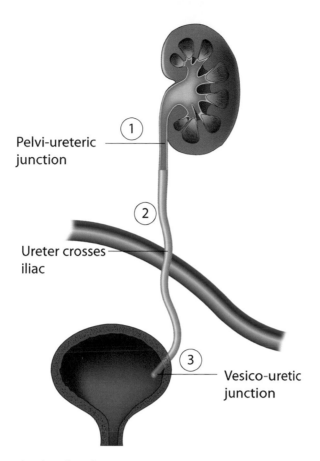

Pelvi-ureteric
junction ─── ①

Ureter crosses ── ②
iliac

③ ── Vesico-uretic
junction

Figure 13.1.1 Obstruction sites of renal stones.

infection along with obstruction, or obstruction of a solitary kidney, urgent treatment is required. This can be in the form of insertion of a percutaneous nephrostomy tube or retrograde insertion of a ureteric stent.

Ureteric stones

Ureteric stones <**5 mm** in diameter will often pass spontaneously and are managed non-pharmacologically unless there is evidence of infection or anatomical abnormality. Management may also include expulsive therapy in the form of an alpha-blocker (e.g. tamsulosin), which has been shown to increase stone expulsion in stones ≤5 mm in the distal ureter.

Ureteric stones >**5 mm** with no evidence of infection and not in a solitary kidney can be managed conservatively with close observation and repeated imaging along with urine sieving to check for stone passage. Larger ureteric stones and stones that do not appear to be moving down the ureter may require surgical intervention with ureteroscopy, stone fragmentation and removal, using a small telescope usually along with a laser to break up the stone. Occasionally, extracorporeal shock wave lithotripsy (ESWL; the use of special sound waves focussed on the stone to break it up) can be used, but this is not usually very effective for stones in the ureter.

Renal stones

Stones within the **kidney** (rather than in the ureter) will often cause no symptoms but at times can cause pain, infection and bleeding and pose the risk of dropping into the ureter, causing renal/ureteric colic.

Renal stones can be managed in various ways depending on their size, position and composition.

- Minimally invasive options:
  - Shock wave lithotripsy: Shatters stones but may cause infection and slight renal injury; CI in pregnancy
  - Flexible ureterorenoscopy: Inserting a flexible telescope up the ureter into the kidney collecting system, breaking the stone with a laser and collecting stone fragments with a small basket device
  - Percutaneous nephrolithotomy: Keyhole surgery to remove stones
  - Ureteroscopy: Ureteroscope passed through the ureter to remove stones and a stent inserted
- Very occasionally laparoscopic or even open surgery is used to remove stones if the other modalities have failed

Chronic disease

Fifty percent of patients will have another renal stone within the next decade, so chronic disease management is focussed on preventing stone formation.

General preventative measures:

- Increase fluid intake (aim for 2–3 litres/day)
- Eat a balanced diet
- Reduce salt intake
- Maintain a healthy weight

Specific preventative measures:

- Calcium stones (oxalate and phosphate):
  - Avoid excessive dietary intake of animal protein, sodium and oxalate-rich products (rhubarb, chocolate, strawberries)
  - Avoid vitamin D supplementation
  - Bendroflumethiazide may help if patient has hypercalciuria
- Struvite: If chronic UTI present (e.g. *Proteus*), treat with prevention of infections
- Uric acid: Avoid excessive dietary intake of urate-rich products (beer, liver, kidney, fish)

13.2 BENIGN PROSTATIC ENLARGEMENT AND LOWER URINARY TRACT SYMPTOMS

DEFINITION

Benign prostatic enlargement (BPE) is an increase in the size of the prostate gland in the absence of malignancy. This can lead to lower urinary tract symptoms that can be divided into storage, voiding and postmicturition symptoms.

EPIDEMIOLOGY

Over 50% of men 50–79 years of age have lower urinary tract symptoms, increasing to over 90% for men in their 90s.

AETIOLOGY

There are many possible causes of lower urinary tract symptoms (LUTS), including BPE. The aetiology of BPE is unclear but there are a number of potential risk factors for its development. Risk factors include increasing age, family history and circulating androgens (BPE does not occur in boys who have been castrated). Afro-Caribbean men are also more likely to develop BPE. Other potential risk factors include obesity, reduced physical activity, diabetes and increased alcohol intake.

PATHOLOGY

BPE is due to stromal and epithelial hyperplasia (increased number of cells) and hypertrophy (increased size of cells). The transitional zone (innermost zone surrounding the urethra) enlarges, compressing the prostatic urethra and leading to symptoms. This is in contrast to prostate cancer, which affects the peripheral zone of the prostate and tends to cause urinary symptoms only when it is more advanced. Testosterone and its active metabolite dihydrotestosterone, which is converted from testosterone by 5-alpha-reductase, are necessary for the development of the prostate and are a target for treatment.

CLINICAL PRESENTATION

LUTS can be divided into storage, voiding and postmicturition symptoms:

Storage symptoms: Urgency, frequency of micturition, nocturia, urgency urinary incontinence.

Voiding symptoms: Hesitancy, intermittency, slow stream, straining, terminal dribble.

Postmicturition symptoms: Postmicturition dribble, sensation of incomplete emptying.

Patients may also present with complications of BPE (10% present this way):

- Recurrent UTI
- Acute retention of urine
- Overflow incontinence
- Obstructive nephropathy

EXAMINATION

This should include a full abdominal examination (look for the presence of a distended bladder and palpable kidneys) and in medical school examinations may include performing a digital rectal examination (DRE) on a model that may reveal a smooth, enlarged prostate.

If you have a simulated station where a patient with BPE presents in acute urinary retention, then you should also examine for perineal sensation to rule out cauda equina syndrome.

INVESTIGATIONS

Bedside:

- Urinalysis: Specifically midstream urine (dipstick for infection and glucose), MC&S
- Request a drinking and voiding diary for 3 days, asking the patient to document time and volume of urine
- Request completion of a symptom score such as the International Prostate Symptom Score (IPSS)
- Flow rate and postmicturition USS to check for residual volume of urine left in the bladder after voiding (>100 mL is abnormal)
- Bloods: FBC (infection), PSA (↑ levels may indicate prostate cancer; perform before DRE as can ↑ levels – see Section 13.3), U&Es (check for obstructive nephropathy), blood glucose (exclude diabetes)

DIFFERENTIAL DIAGNOSIS

There can be many different causes of LUTS in addition to BPE, including UTI, distal ureteric stone (see Section 13.1), urethral stricture, detrusor under/overactivity, neurogenic bladder dysfunction and bladder tumours. Certain medical conditions should also be considered especially with urinary frequency, such as diabetes mellitus, diabetes insipidus, hypercalcaemia and uraemia.

MANAGEMENT

BPE may present acutely with complications:

- Recurrent UTI:
  - Defined as two or more episodes in a 3-month period
  - Admit to hospital if systemically unwell or showing signs of urosepsis (shock, tachypnoea, vomiting)
  - Advise sufficient fluid intake to avoid dehydration to reduce the risk of UTI
  - Simple analgesia and antibiotic treatment with trimethoprim or nitrofurantoin for 7 days
  - Arrange 2-week wait referral for bladder cancer if ≥60 with unexplained recurrent UTI

- Acute urinary retention:
  - Rule out cauda equina syndrome
  - Encourage voiding with analgesia and standing
  - If unsuccessful, catheterise the patient

Chronic disease
Non-pharmacological

- Educate about the condition
- Use a drinking and voiding diary to assess the type of fluid consumption and pattern of voiding
- Diet advice: Reduce caffeine and alcohol intake, prudent fluid intake, prevention of constipation
- Bladder training (e.g. increase time between voiding)
- Containment products (pads, waterproof pants) and consider referral to the continence team
- Perform an IPSS to guide need for medical management and response to treatment

Pharmacological

- Alpha-blockers (**tamsulosin**) → relax prostate smooth muscle. Offer if IPSS ≥8
  - Side effects include postural hypotension and retrograde ejaculation

- If symptoms persist despite treatment with an alpha-blocker (and there is not a significant postvoid residual) then consider adding an antimuscarinic medication (e.g. **tolterodine**). Side effects include dryness and constipation and potentially urinary retention
- 5-alpha-reductase inhibitors (**finasteride**) → inhibit conversion of testosterone to dihydrotestosterone. Offer if patient has LUTS and a prostate estimated to be >30 g or a PSA ≥1.4 ng/mL and a high risk of progression (older man, poor urine flow, high symptoms score and high PSA). Side effects include erectile dysfunction
- **Urinary catheterisation** can be used and can be intermittent, indwelling urethral or indwelling suprapubic

Surgical

Surgery is usually required for a large prostate/failure to respond to medical therapy.

- Transurethral resection of the prostate (TURP)
- Transurethral vaporisation of the prostate (TUVP)
- Transurethral laser enucleation of the prostate
- Open prostatectomy for extremely large prostates (very rarely performed now due to the success of less invasive modalities)

13.3 PROSTATE CANCER

DEFINITION

Prostate cancer is a primary malignant neoplasm of the prostate gland.

EPIDEMIOLOGY

Prostate cancer is the most common type of cancer in men (accounting for >25% of new cancer diagnoses in men, around 130 every day or over 47,000 per year in the UK). It is the second most common cause of cancer death in males in the UK (>11,500 per year). One in eight men will be diagnosed with prostate cancer in their lifetime.

AETIOLOGY

Genetic, hormonal and viral factors are thought to play a part in its development. Risk factors include age, family history, Afro-Caribbean ethnicity and high fat, meat and alcohol intake. There are a number of genetic mutations associated with prostate cancer that can differ greatly in growth rates and metastatic potential.

PATHOLOGY

The majority of prostate cancers are **adenocarcinomas**. These affect the outer zone of the prostate gland.

Prostate cancer metastases can spread to lymph nodes early in the disease process (obturator lymph nodes).

It also tends to spread predominantly to the bones, producing **osteosclerotic** lesions on x-ray (usually metastases cause osteolytic lesions).

Causes of a raised PSA

- Prostate cancer
- Benign prostatic enlargement
- Prostatitis
- Urinary tract infection
- Recent ejaculation
- Recent vigorous exercise

CLINICAL PRESENTATION

Often asymptomatic – many prostate cancers are found via an incidental raised PSA on blood tests.

There is currently no formal screening programme in the UK (PSA + DRE unreliable, MRI is expensive/inaccurate).

NICE recommends suspecting prostate cancer in men with weight loss/anorexia and any of the following:

Localised disease:

- Lower urinary tract symptoms (hesitancy, poor stream, nocturia, terminal dribbling, frequency)
- Recurrent UTI

Locally invasive disease (localised to the prostate capsule and seminal vesicles):

- Haematuria, dysuria, incontinence
- Suprapubic pain
- Erectile dysfunction

Metastatic spread:

- Lower back pain or bone pain
- Pathological fractures
- Renal failure secondary to obstruction

EXAMINATION

Digital rectal examination (DRE) may reveal a hard, irregular prostate – in your final examinations this will most likely be incorporated by using a model.

NICE Guidelines 2017

Refer the patient urgently on the suspected cancer pathway (2-week wait) if:

- DRE examination reveals a hard, nodular prostate
- PSA levels are above the age-specific reference range. For men 50–69 this is 3.0 ng/mL or higher

---

INVESTIGATIONS

Bedside: Urinalysis and MC&S (presence of haematuria, UTI).

Bloods: FBC (anaemia), U&Es (renal function), LFTs ($\uparrow$ ALP), bone profile ($\uparrow$ Ca^{2+}), PSA ($\uparrow$) (see box).

Imaging:

- Multi-parametric MRI can potentially reduce the need for prostate biopsies and can help targeting of prostate biopsies
- Bone scan can be used to identify bone metastases

Invasive: Prostate biopsies. These can either be performed as transrectal ultrasound-guided biopsies (up to 45% of tumours may be missed) or transperineal template-guided biopsies.

DIFFERENTIAL DIAGNOSIS

The main differential diagnosis is BPE (see Section 13.2). and UTI. UTI must be excluded prior to PSA testing.

GLEASON SCORE

The Gleason score is used to classify whether a prostate tumour is low, intermediate or high grade. It is calculated using 10–12 sections of the prostate taken during biopsy and gives a score from 2 to 10.

Low grade ≤ 6; intermediate grade 7; high grade ≥ 8.

Table 13.3.1 Risk stratification for localised prostate cancer (i.e. not locally advanced or metastatic)

Risk of progression	PSA level (ng/mL)		Gleason score		Clinical stage
Low	<10	And	≤6	And	T1-T2a
Intermediate	10–20	Or	7	Or	T2b
High	>20	Or	8–10	Or	≥T2c

NICE has published a risk stratification for men according to PSA levels, Gleason score and TNM clinical stage (*Table 13.3.1*).

MANAGEMENT

Management is primarily determined by the stage of the disease with different treatment for localised, locally advanced and metastatic disease (*Table 13.3.2*).

Localised disease

Management is aimed to be curative and prevent progression.

Low-risk disease:

- Watchful waiting if patient is asymptomatic and has a life expectancy <10 years. This involves monitoring PSA and symptoms
- Active surveillance for patients suitable for curative treatment and life expectancy >10 years. This involves regular PSA blood testing, DRE and possible repeat MRI or prostate biopsies
- Radical prostatectomy now usually performed as a robotically-assisted laparoscopic operation
- External beam radiotherapy (EBR)
- Brachytherapy (insertion of radioactive seeds into the prostate)

Intermediate-risk disease:

- Radical prostatectomy
- EBR, usually with androgen deprivation therapy before and during treatment (see next section)
- Active surveillance (only in very select lower risk patients)

High-risk disease:

- EBR with androgen deprivation therapy before, during and for 2–3 years after treatment
- Radical prostatectomy but this carries a significant risk of positive surgical margins

Locally advanced disease

Management is again aimed to be curative and prevent progression.

- EBR with androgen deprivation for 2–3 years
- Radical prostatectomy, only really in T3a disease, and patients need to be informed that they may need additional treatments such as radiotherapy

Metastatic disease

Management is palliative with the hope of long-term control of the cancer/symptoms.

- Androgen deprivation therapy, usually with an LHRH agonist (e.g. goserelin [Zoladex], see box) or antagonist (e.g. degarelix). Bilateral orchidectomy is a surgical option
- Patients who are fit enough can have chemotherapy (e.g. docetaxel) or abiraterone (which blocks tumour production of testosterone) along with androgen deprivation therapy

Support

- Educate about the condition
- Discuss support groups (Cancer Research UK, Prostate Cancer UK, Macmillan Cancer Support)
- Management of complications (see next section) and review for symptoms of spinal cord compression

Table 13.3.2 Clinical staging (TNM staging)

Tumour	Nodes	Metastases
T1 Tumour that is not palpable	**N0** No regional lymph node involvement	**M0** No distant metastases
T2 Tumour that is palpable and confined to the prostate (T2a = ≤ half of 1 lobe, T2b = >half of 1 lobe, T2c = involves both lobes)	**N1** Regional lymph node involvement	**M1a** Non-regional lymph nodes
T3 Tumour extends through prostate capsule		**M1b** None
T4 Tumour is fixed/invades adjacent structures other than seminal vesicles, urinary tract, rectum or pelvic wall		**M1c** Other sites

COMPLICATIONS

Hot flushes: Offer cyproterone acetate (an antiandrogen) or medroxyprogesterone.

Fatigue: Aerobic exercise.

Osteoporosis: Bisphosphonates.

Gynaecomastia: If on long-term bicalutamide monotherapy, offer prophylactic radiotherapy.

Urinary symptoms: Bladder retraining + pelvic floor exercises.

Erectile dysfunction: Offer sildenafil.

Goserelin (Zoladex)

GnRH agonist that increases the amount of LH to stimulate testosterone production with the aim to **down-regulate the body's own testosterone production** by negative feedback.

As it initially ↑ testosterone levels, it can cause worsening of symptoms, so an antiandrogen is often co-prescribed (e.g. bicalutamide).

UROLOGY: QUESTIONS

13.1 RENAL/URETERIC STONES

1. Which is the most common type of renal stone by composition?

2. Where are the three locations where renal stones usually obstruct?

3. What management options are available for renal stones <5 mm without evidence of obstruction or anatomical abnormality?

13.2 BENIGN PROSTATIC ENLARGEMENT AND LOWER URINARY TRACT SYMPTOMS

1. Name three voiding and three storage lower urinary tract symptoms that patients with BPE may present with.

2. Describe the pharmacological treatment options for BPE and their mechanism of action.

3. What surgical options are there for managing BPH?

13.3 PROSTATE CANCER

1. Prostate cancers are adenocarcinomas that generally affect which part of the prostate gland?

2. What are the causes for a raised PSA?

3. Describe the three main stages of prostate cancer and possible treatment options for them.

CHAPTER 14

Vascular Surgery

14.1 PERIPHERAL ARTERIAL DISEASE

DEFINITION

Peripheral arterial disease is a term used to describe narrowing or occlusion of peripheral arteries, which manifests in a reduction in blood supply to the lower limbs. Limb ischaemia can occur acutely or chronically.

EPIDEMIOLOGY

In the UK, 20% of the age 55–75 population have evidence of lower extremity peripheral arterial disease, of which 5% have symptoms. Chronic limb ischaemia is much more common than acute limb ischaemia.

Risk factors for the development of peripheral arterial disease can be split into modifiable and non-modifiable.

Modifiable risk factors: Hypertension, smoking, ↑ cholesterol, diabetes, obesity, sedentary lifestyle.

Non-modifiable risk factors: Family history, increasing age, sex (M > F until menopause, when M = F).

The principal risk factor for the development of peripheral arterial disease (in >50s) is **smoking**.

AETIOLOGY/PATHOLOGY

Peripheral arterial disease is predominantly caused by **atherosclerosis** and subsequent narrowing of the arteries supplying the lower limb. Rarely, it can be due to pathologies such as vasculitis or vessel entrapment.

Acute limb ischaemia is most commonly caused by **thrombosis/embolus** over an atherosclerotic plaque.

CLINICAL PRESENTATION

Acute limb ischaemia presents with acute changes in the distal limb that can be remembered by the **6Ps** (see box).

> ### The 6 Ps of an acutely ischaemic limb
>
> **P**ain
> **P**allor
> **P**araesthesia
> **P**aralysis
> **P**erishingly cold
> **P**ulselessness

If the acute limb ischaemia is due to an embolus, the onset is often acute (seconds to minutes) with profound ischaemia. Due to the embolic nature, there may not be a history of chronic limb ischaemia and the pulses in the other leg may be normal. If the acute limb ischaemia is due to thrombosis, the onset is insidious (hours to days), often with a history of chronic limb ischaemia (e.g. claudication and weak peripheral pulses in both limbs).

Chronic limb ischaemia typically presents as a progressively worsening cramp-like pain on walking (**intermittent claudication**), typically felt in the foot, calf or buttock, which is relieved by rest. Symptoms may also be worse at night (due to a fall in blood pressure and therefore a reduced perfusion). Patients may also present with non-healing wounds over the lower limb.

EXAMINATION

A peripheral arterial examination involves a whole-body examination.

Upper limb: Inspect the upper limb for skin changes (pale, pink), ischaemic changes (gangrene) and for evidence of underlying risk factors such as tar staining and tendon xanthomata. Feel for temperature, capillary refill and radial and brachial pulses and take blood pressure in both arms.

Face: Look for corneal arcus, xanthelasma (↑ lipids) and central cyanosis and feel the carotid pulses.

Abdomen: Inspect for scars and pulsation of aorta. Palpate and auscultate for AAA.

Lower limb: Inspect the skin for colour changes, scars (previous CABG venous grafting). Feel for temperature, capillary refill and pulses (starting proximally at the popliteal, posterior tibial, dorsalis pedis). Squeeze the calves, looking for evidence of tenderness (suggestive of critical ischaemia).

Special tests: **Buerger's test** (for reperfusion time):

- With the patient lying supine, lift their leg until the heel becomes pale
- The angle at which the heel becomes pale is Buerger's angle. If the heel does not go pale, then this is a normal test
- Keep the pale heel in the air for 30 seconds
- Ask the patient to sit up and hang their legs over the side of the bed and watch their feet
- A positive sequala typically shows pallor, then reactive hyperaemia (redness), which implies significant peripheral arterial disease

It is good practice to state that you would ideally perform a full cardiovascular examination and sensory assessment of the lower limb followed by a Doppler ultrasound for peripheral pulses.

INVESTIGATIONS

Bedside: ECG (detect any cardiovascular changes), urine dipstick (looking for glucose [DM])

Bloods: FBC (anaemia causing pallor), U&Es (peripheral arterial disease associated with renal artery stenosis and CKD), blood glucose/HbA1c (DM), lipids (↑)

Imaging: USS Doppler (detect peripheral pulses). Ankle-brachial pressure index (ABPI) to confirm diagnosis

An ABPI ratio of <0.9 indicates the presence of peripheral arterial disease (normal range 1.0–1.2)

Intermittent claudication is associated with an ABPI of between 0.5–0.9

An ABPI of <0.5 is suggestive of critical limb ischaemia

An ABPI of ≥1.3 is associated with hardening of arterial vessels in conditions such as renal failure or diabetes, which may cause peripheral arterial disease

DIFFERENTIAL DIAGNOSIS

The differential diagnosis for peripheral arterial disease includes venous claudication, sciatica, osteoarthritis, peripheral neuropathy, popliteal artery entrapment, spinal canal claudication, fibromuscular dysplasia and Buerger's disease.

MANAGEMENT
Acute limb ischaemia

If acute limb ischaemia is suspected, emergency assessment and treatment are required by vascular surgeons.

Surgical options depend on the location of the lesion, comorbidities and risk of treatment.

Surgical options include:

- Surgical embolectomy
- Endovascular revascularisation
- Percutaneous thrombolytic therapy
- Amputation of the limb

Chronic limb Ischaemia
Non-pharmacological

- Manage lifestyle risk factors:
  - Stop smoking
  - Diet and weight management
  - Exercise (NICE recommends offering a **supervised exercise programme** to all people with intermittent claudication, or unsupervised exercise of 30 minutes 3–5 times per week, where patients exercise until the onset of symptoms, then rest to recover)
- Patients need to inform the DVLA if they hold a bus, coach or HGV license; car/motorcycle drivers do not

Pharmacological

- Symptomatic treatment: **Naftidrofuryl oxalate** (vasodilator) can be prescribed if exercise has not led to an improvement and the patient does not want to be referred for surgery
- Managing cardiovascular risk (secondary prevention):
  - **Antiplatelet** treatment: **Clopidogrel** is the preferred antiplatelet
  - **Lipid** modification: High-dose statin (e.g. **atorvastatin** 80 mg) (see box)
  - **Hypertension** management (see Section 1.3)
  - Optimise management of **diabetes** if applicable

Surgical

- If a patient has not had satisfactory improvement from an exercise programme, then they can be referred to vascular surgery for consideration of surgical intervention. Options include:
  - Angioplasty
  - Bypass surgery

Investigations and monitoring for initiation of statin therapy

Baseline tests

- Lipid measurement
- Creatine kinase (CK)
- LFTs
- Renal function (CKD may need a ↓ dose)
- HbA1c
- TFTs

Monitoring

- Check lipids at 3 months
- Check LFTs at 3 and 12 months
- Review bloods annually

Adverse effects: If a patient develops unexplained muscle symptoms, check CK. Consider stopping the statin if muscle symptoms cannot be tolerated or if serum CK level is five times the upper limit of normal.

14.2 VENOUS INSUFFICIENCY

VARICOSE VEINS

Definition

Varicose veins are tortuous and dilated superficial leg veins.

Epidemiology

Varicose veins are common, found in between 10%–20% of men and 25%–33% of women. Risk factors for developing them include age, parity, obesity and occupation (a lot of standing).

Aetiology/Pathology

Varicose veins occur because of incompetent valves in a vein that cause a reflux of blood distally. Blood flows backwards from the deep venous system to the superficial venous system, causing an increased backpressure. Increased pressure causes a widening and leakage of further valves. Blood pools, and the superficial veins dilate.

The majority of varicose veins are primary. Secondary varicose veins occur due to deep vein thrombosis (DVT), pelvic tumours, pregnancy or an arteriovenous fistula.

Clinical presentation

Patients may present after noticing the dilated, superficial veins on their lower limb and may be concerned. Alternatively, they may have symptoms of heaviness or aching in the leg (worse on standing, improved by elevating). Patients may present with a complication of varicose veins (see box).

Complications of varicose veins

Haemorrhage

Varicose eczema

Venous ulceration

Thrombophlebitis

Oedema

Lipodermatosclerosis

Haemosiderin deposition

Examination

Examining for varicose veins is not routinely included in a CVS examination. The steps are outlined here:

Inspection: Comment on the distribution of the varicose veins and which veins may be affected (the long saphenous vein runs up the medial side of the leg whereas the short saphenous vein runs up the lateral side).

Look for evidence of skin changes: Venous eczema, haemosiderin deposition (brown patches from damaged leaky vessels), lipdodermatosclerosis (redness from inflammation of subcutaneous fat), venous ulcers

(which are typically painless and occur around the medial malleoli – compared to arterial ulcers, which are painful and occur around the lateral malleoli).

Palpation: Palpate the varicosities and comment on tenderness and hardness (suggestive of phlebitis). Palpate the saphenofemoral junction (5 cm below and medial to femoral pulse) and check a cough impulse (suggestive of a saphena varix). Perform the **Trendelenburg test**: lift the leg as high as possible to empty the veins and place a tourniquet over the saphenofemoral junction. While maintaining pressure over the junction, ask the patient to stand and witness whether the varicosities refill. If the varicosities refill, it suggests the incompetent valve lies below the level of the saphenofemoral junction. Repeat the test, moving the tourniquet down 3 cm each time until the varicosities do not refill to identify the region of incompetence.

Percussion: Tap distally on the varicosities and feel an impulse proximally (normal) and then reverse. If you can feel an impulse proximally when tapping distally, this suggests incompetent veins.

Complete your examination by completing an abdominal and pelvic examination (looking for masses).

Investigations

Varicose veins are a clinical diagnosis, and investigations are used to rule out secondary causes (e.g. D-dimer for DVT, abdominal/pelvic USS looking for masses) if suggested by the clinical scenario. ABPI should be completed to exclude peripheral arterial disease before recommending compression hosiery.

Chronic disease management

Non-pharmacological

- Reassure the patient that varicose veins are common
- Recommend lifestyle advice if necessary (lose weight, physical activity, avoid triggers)
- If symptoms are troublesome, compression stockings can be offered after a satisfactory ABPI

Surgical

If there are complications or troublesome symptoms not controlled by compression stockings, then vascular surgery can be considered. Options include surgical removal, ligation, foam sclerotherapy and endothermal methods.

DEEP VEIN THROMBOSIS

Definition

Deep vein thrombosis (DVT) is a formation of a thrombus in a deep vein, usually in the legs, which either partially or completely obstructs blood flow. The most serious complication of a DVT is a pulmonary embolism.

Epidemiology

DVTs have an incidence of 1 in 1000 people in the UK. Risk factors for developing a DVT include previous DVT, malignancy, increasing age, obesity, heart failure, thrombophilia, vascular wall trauma (e.g. vasculitis), immobility, hormone treatment (e.g. HRT), pregnancy, dehydration and recent surgery.

Aetiology/Pathology

The formation of a DVT is associated with **Virchow's triad** – three states that predispose to DVT formation:

- Endothelial damage: Exposes subendothelial collagen, which gives platelets a surface to bind to
- Stasis: Increases the likelihood of coagulation factors coming into contact with damaged surfaces and each other
- Hypercoagulability: Shifts the coagulation pathway towards thrombus formation

Clinical presentation

A DVT classically presents with **pain** and **swelling** in one leg. It is possible to get bilateral DVTs, but very unlikely. It is important to ascertain any risk factors for the development of a DVT in the history (Table 14.2.1).

Examination

The affected leg may have signs of venous distension (**prominent veins**), changes to skin colour (**redness**), and be **warm** and **tender** to touch. A **tape measure** should be used to compare the size of one calf to the other. As well as confirming the typical signs of a DVT, examination should also aim to exclude other conditions that may present in a similar fashion, e.g. cellulitis (look for evidence of a break in the skin – patients may also have a raised temperature), pitting oedema (usually bilateral and may have signs of right-sided heart failure/renal failure/hepatic failure), venous insufficiency, acute limb ischaemia (see Section 14.1), a ruptured Baker's cyst (check in the popliteal fossa), compartment syndrome and physical trauma.

Investigations

Bedside: Calf measurement, urine dip (renal failure)

Bloods: D-dimer (↑), FBC (infection), U&Es (renal failure), LFTs

Imaging: USS (confirms diagnosis)

Differential diagnosis

The differential diagnosis for a DVT includes physical trauma (e.g. fracture/calf strain), thrombophlebitis, venous insufficiency, acute limb ischaemia, vasculitis, ruptured Baker's cyst, cellulitis and compartment syndrome.

Management

Centres may recommend performing a **Wells score** in patients suspected to have a DVT (Table 14.2.1). If the score is ≥2 then a DVT is likely and a proximal leg vein USS should be carried out to confirm. If the score is 1 or less, then a D-dimer blood test should be performed. If D-dimer is raised, a proximal leg vein USS should be performed. If, in either instance, the USS cannot be performed within 4 hours, LMWH should be administered. Once the USS has confirmed the diagnosis, interim therapeutic anticoagulation should be started.

Depending on the person's preferences and comorbities, the options for anticoagulation include either:

- Apixaban or Rivaroxaban
- LMWH for 5 days followed by Dabigatran or Edoxaban
- LMWH for 5 days concurrently with Warfarin

Anticoagulation treatment is usually continued for three months. If the DVT was considered to be 'unprovoked', then NICE recommend extending anticoagulation treatment for up to 6 months. Furthermore, unprovoked DVTs should be investigated for underlying malignancy with an examination, CXR and blood tests (FBC, bone profile, LFTs) and urinalysis.

REFERENCE

https://cks.nice.org.uk/topics/deep-vein-thrombosis/management/management/

Table 14.2.1 Wells score for DVT risk factors

Clinical feature	Score
Active cancer (ongoing treatment or <6 months)	1
Paralysis or recent plaster immobilisation	1
Bedridden for 3 days or major surgery <12 weeks	1
Localised tenderness along deep veins	1
Entire leg swollen	1
Calf swelling at least 3 cm greater than asymptomatic side	1
Pitting oedema only on symptomatic leg	1
Superficial (non-varicose) veins	1
Previous documented DVT	1
Alternative diagnosis is at least as likely as DVT	−2

14.3 ABDOMINAL AORTIC ANEURYSM

DEFINITION

An aneurysm is a permanent and irreversible dilation of a blood vessel by at least 50% of the normal expected diameter. The most important aneurysm to know about for finals is an abdominal aortic aneurysm (AAA).

EPIDEMIOLOGY

AAAs are more common in men (6:1) and have a prevalence of around 4% in men aged 65–74 in the UK.

Risk factors for an AAA include smoking, hypertension, male sex, hyperlipidaemia and family history.

Factors that predispose AAAs to rupture include increasing diameter, COPD, smoking, hypertension, family history and inflammation within the aneurysm wall. If an AAA ruptures, without rapid surgical or endovascular treatment there is almost 100% mortality within 3 days.

AETIOLOGY/PATHOLOGY

Most AAAs are thought to be caused secondary to an atherosclerotic process in the aorta. A minority of AAAs are caused by trauma, inflammatory diseases (vasculitis), connective tissue disorders and infection (e.g. endocarditis).

The majority of AAAs (90%) emerge below the renal arteries.

CLINICAL PRESENTATION

Most AAAs are discovered as an incidental finding on abdominal examination or on imaging (x-ray/USS)

through the National Abdominal Aortic Aneurysm Screening Programme (NAAASP; Figure 14.3.1).

Possible presenting symptoms for an unruptured AAA include back pain, abdominal pain, or loin/groin pain due to the pressure effect on local structures. Other presenting symptoms include distal embolisation producing features similar to peripheral arterial disease.

If an AAA ruptures, this is a surgical emergency. Patients will present with hypovolaemic shock ± syncope ± severe central abdominal pain radiating to the back ± pulsatile mass in the abdomen.

EXAMINATION

Examination for an AAA should be included in an abdominal examination and peripheral arterial examination.

INVESTIGATIONS

Bedside: ECG

Bloods: FBC (↓Hb), clotting screen, renal function (hypovolaemia compromising renal function), cross-match (if surgery planned), inflammatory markers (if inflammatory cause suspected)

Imaging: USS abdomen (can confirm aneurysm but not exclude rupture), AXR (may show calcified aorta), CT (can confirm the diagnosis of a ruptured AAA in stable patients)

Invasive: MRI angiography

DIFFERENTIAL DIAGNOSIS

AAA may mimic a number of conditions presenting as abdominal pain and therefore any condition that can

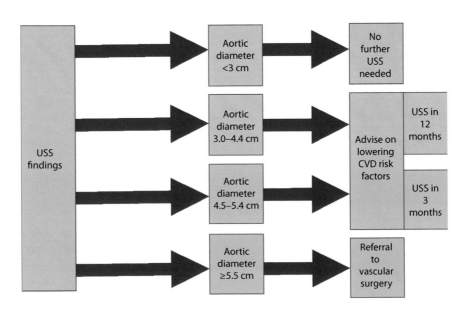

Figure 14.3.1 Unruptured AAA surveillance.

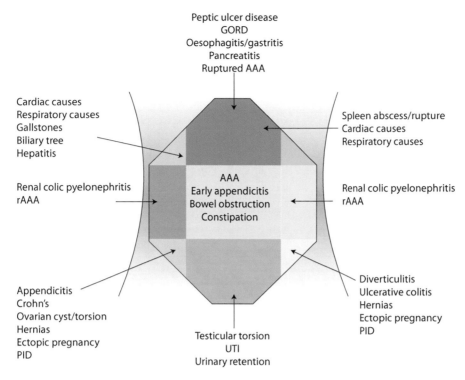

Figure 14.3.2 Differential diagnosis of the acute abdomen.

present as an acute abdomen should be included in your differential (Figure 14.3.2).

The Royal College of Emergency Medicine states that a clinical diagnosis of a ruptured AAA can be made:

- In patients >50 years of age presenting with acute-onset abdominal/back pain AND hypotension
- In patients with known AAA symptoms of either abdominal/back pain OR hypotension/collapse

MANAGEMENT
Acute ruptured AAA

A ruptured AAA is a surgical emergency and management should follow an **ABCDE approach**.

Resuscitation should be performed and IV access gained as early as possible with bloods taken for crossmatch.

Theatre should be attended immediately and not delayed for investigation findings.

Due to the severity of the hypovolaemic shock in some cases, surgery may be required to stem the bleeding rather than by fluid resuscitation.

Unruptured AAA

Once an unruptured AAA is discovered, the management predominantly depends on its size (see next).

The NAAASP offers all men >65 years a single abdominal USS. Men >65 years old can self-refer. If on USS assessment:

- The aortic diameter is <3 cm, no further USS are planned
- The aortic diameter is found to be 3.0–4.4 cm, non-pharmacological management is offered (Figure 14.3.1) with a further scan in 12 months
- The aortic diameter is 4.5–5.4 cm, non-pharmacological management is offered with a further scan in 3 months
- The aortic diameter is ≥5.5 cm, the patient is referred to vascular surgery due to increased risk of rupture

Non-pharmacological management for lowering cardiovascular risk factors include:

- Lifestyle changes (stop smoking, regular exercise, losing weight, healthy eating)
- Appropriate cardiovascular prevention medications:
  - Hypertension management
  - Lipid management
  - Antiplatelet medication

VASCULAR SURGERY: QUESTIONS

14.1 PERIPHERAL ARTERIAL DISEASE

1. What are the risk factors for developing peripheral arterial disease?
2. What are the presenting features of an acute ischaemic limb?
3. What management options are available for treating peripheral arterial disease?

14.2 VENOUS INSUFFICIENCY

1. What are the complications of varicose veins?
2. What are the surgical options for treating varicose veins?

3. Name three risk factors for the development of a deep vein thrombosis.
4. What are the treatment options for an unprovoked DVT?

14.3 ABDOMINAL AORTIC ANEURYSM

1. Where do the majority of abdominal aortic aneurysms occur?
2. At what aneurysm size are patients referred to vascular surgery following screening?
3. What non-pharmacological management options are recommended for patients with an abdominal aortic aneurysm?

CHAPTER 15

Ear, Nose and Throat

15.1 VERTIGO

DEFINITION
Vertigo is defined as an illusion of movement that a person's surroundings are spinning or rotating in the absence of any physical movement.

EPIDEMIOLOGY
Prevalence estimate for true vertigo in the general population is around 5%, with the most common cause of vertigo being benign position paroxysmal vertigo (BPPV).

AETIOLOGY/PATHOLOGY
Vertigo can be caused by a number of conditions. An important distinction to make is the difference between 'true' vertigo and general dizziness/unsteadiness that may have a cardiovascular aetiology, e.g. vertebrobasilar insufficiency, which occurs when elderly patients rotate their neck leading to a temporary decrease in blood flow to the posterior circulation in the brain. It is most commonly due to an atherosclerotic process.

True vertigo can be caused by:

Benign position paroxysmal vertigo (BPPV): Possibly caused by loose otoliths/otoconia in the labyrinth.

Generalised age-related disequilibrium (GARD): Occurs due to age-related changes in the vestibular system.

Ménière's disease: Triad of unilateral deafness, vertigo and tinnitus and fullness in the ear. Due to dilation of endolymphatic spaces.

Acoustic neuroma: Benign neoplasm of the superior vestibular nerve. Presents with a slow onset of symptoms.

Vestibular migraine: Vertigo secondary to a migraine, often with a family history of migraines.

Acute vestibular neuronitis: Inflammation of the vestibular nerve that classically occurs secondary to a URTI and normal hearing.

Acute labyrinthitis: Inflammation of the labyrinth that classically occurs secondary to a viral URTI.

Central lesions (such as multiple sclerosis/stroke/tumour).

CLINICAL PRESENTATION
The causes of vertigo can be distinguished by the length of the vertigo attacks and the presence of any associated symptoms (such as nausea, deafness, tinnitus, VII nerve problems and recent viral symptoms).

Length of attacks
Episodic vertigo lasting seconds to minutes: Consider BPPV.

Episodic vertigo lasting minutes to hours: Consider Ménière's disease, vestibular migraine or GARD.

Vertigo lasting >24 hours: Consider a central lesion (such as a stroke, multiple sclerosis or tumour) or a peripheral lesion such as acute vestibular neuronitis or acute labyrinthitis.

Other signs in the history that will guide you towards the diagnosis include:

- Very short attacks which occur with sudden changes in posture (such as turning head at night): BPPV
- Attacks that occur with unilateral hearing loss, tinnitus and a sense of fullness in the ear: Ménière's
- Attacks that occur with a preceding aura associated with a headache: Vestibular migraine
- Prolonged constant attacks of vertigo without hearing loss: Acute vestibular neuronitis
- Prolonged constant attacks of vertigo **with** hearing loss: Acute labyrinthitis

EXAMINATION
Examination should include a neurological examination looking for cerebellar signs (such as nystagmus).

Sitting and standing blood pressure should be measured to exclude a postural cause of dizziness and to help distinguish between dizziness and vertigo.

If BPPV is suspected the Dix–Hallpike manoeuvre can be performed:

- The patient is positioned sitting on the bed with their legs stretched in front of them, so when lying flat, their head will hang off the top edge of the bed.
- Left and right sides are tested in turn.
- Turn the patient's head 45 degrees towards you while holding both sides of the head and quickly lie them flat in one motion so that their head is hanging down off the end of the bed.
- Ask the patient to keep their eyes open and observe any nystagmus.
- A positive test occurs when there is nystagmus following the change in head position. The patient will often report a recurrence of their vertigo symptoms.
- If the test is positive, the Epley manoeuvre can be performed once the nystagmus has settled.

INVESTIGATIONS
Bedside: BP.

Imaging: If a stroke or MS is suspected as a cause, then a CT or MRI should be performed, respectively.

Before diagnosing Ménière's disease, an MRI should be performed to exclude an acoustic neuroma.

DIFFERENTIAL DIAGNOSIS

Table 15.1.1 presents the differential diagnoses for vertigo.

MANAGEMENT

If a patient has sudden attacks of vertigo, consider the risks of swimming and operating dangerous machinery. Advise patients who have sudden attacks of vertigo to inform the DVLA.

Menière's disease

Non-pharmacological

- Educate the patient regarding the risks before driving, operating dangerous machinery, using ladders or going swimming
- Encourage the patient to move around after an attack (vestibular rehabilitation)

- Sound therapy, relaxation techniques and avoiding silent environments for tinnitus
- Reassure the patient that an acute attack of vertigo will normally settle within 1–2 days in most people

Pharmacological

- Short-term (7–14 days) prochlorperazine or an antihistamine (cinnarizine, cyclizine)
- Prevention of attacks: Trial of betahistine (16 mg TDS) and low-salt diet

Surgical

Intratympanic ototoxic drugs (aminoglycosides) can be injected directly into the middle ear after a procedure has been performed to cut through the tympanic membrane.

Table 15.1.1 Differential diagnoses for vertigo

Condition	Aetiology	Vertigo description	Associated signs/ symptoms	Treatment
Benign paroxysmal positional vertigo (BPPV)	Loose otolith	Episodic vertigo Lasts seconds Triggered by turning head (i.e. in bed)	Nystagmus on Dix–Hallpike	Diagnosis confirmed by observation of nystagmus from the Dix–Hallpike test Epley manoeuvre used for symptomatic relief
Generalised age-related disequilibrium	Age-related changes	Episodic vertigo Lasts minutes–hours Aggravated on standing	No focal neurology or postural hypotension	No recommended medical treatments currently
Vestibular migraine	As for migraine (see Section 6.5)	Episodic vertigo Lasts hours–day Warning aura	Headache Photophobia	As for migraine (see Section 6.5)
Menière's disease	Idiopathic dilatation of endolymphatic spaces	Episodic vertigo Lasts hours No warning	Unilateral hearing loss and tinnitus Sensation of aural pressure	As above
Acoustic neuroma	Benign neoplasm of the vestibular nerve	As for Menière's disease	As for Menière's disease	Referral to ENT for surgery
Acute vestibular neuronitis	Inflammation of the vestibular nerve due to infection	Constant vertigo Lasts days–week	Nausea and vomiting	Cyclizine/ prochlorperazine Usually resolves <3 weeks If last >6 weeks – refer
Acute labyrinthitis	Inflammation of the labyrinth due to infection	As for acute vestibular neuronitis	Nausea and vomiting Hearing impairment	Cyclizine/ prochlorperazine Usually resolves <3 weeks If last >6 weeks – refer

15.2 HEARING LOSS

DEFINITION

Hearing loss is the most common symptom of ear disease and can occur with varying severity. It can be classified as either conductive (where there is a problem of the conductive system of the external or middle ear) or sensorineural (where there is a problem of the cochlear or auditory pathway) or a combination of both.

EPIDEMIOLOGY

Hearing loss is a common presenting complaint in general practice and is most often due to age-related changes (presbyacusis), impacted wax or infection. Rarer, but important, causes to consider include acoustic neuroma and cholesteatoma.

AETIOLOGY/PATHOLOGY

The causes of conductive and sensorineural hearing loss are listed in *Table 15.2.1*.

Presbyacusis: The most common cause in adults. Patients usually >65 years of age with progressive hearing loss ± tinnitus. Thought to be due to the loss of hair cells around the base of the cochlea that can be damaged in older age.

Wax: Impacted wax may occur due to factors preventing extrusion from the ear (e.g. hearing aid/cotton buds).

Otitis media: Febrile patients with inflammation of the middle ear that classically occurs following a URTI.

Menière's disease: Triad of unilateral deafness, vertigo and tinnitus. Due to dilation of endolymphatic spaces.

Acoustic neuroma: Benign neoplasm of the superior vestibular nerve. Presents with a slow onset of symptoms.

Otosclerosis: Autosomal dominant condition that presents with progressive hearing loss, usually due to fixation of the stapes in the oval window. Classically presents in women in their 20s–30s.

CLINICAL PRESENTATION

When clerking a patient with hearing loss, there are several important features to elicit in the history:

- Age: Conditions such as presbyacusis occur in older patients, whereas otosclerosis occurs in younger.
- Timing: Is this an acute aetiology (e.g. tympanic membrane injury) or a progressive (e.g. presbyacusis)?
- Symmetry: Is this hearing loss unilateral or bilateral? Hearing loss is usually bilateral but may be unilateral with either Menière's disease or an acoustic neuroma.
- Associated symptoms: Is there concurrent tinnitus or vertigo (triad is suggestive of Menière's and possibly an acoustic neuroma) or a vesicular rash/facial palsy (suggestive of Ramsay–Hunt syndrome)?

- Risk factors: Has there been a recent URTI (acute otitis media), ototoxic drug use (aminoglycosides/furosemide), frequent air travel (barotrauma) or noise exposure (NIHL)?
- Family history: Could this reveal a congenital cause (e.g. Alport's) or an acquired cause (e.g. otosclerosis)?
- Cranial nerve involvement: Has the patient noticed a change in the function of their cranial nerves (e.g. facial muscles [CN VII], facial sensation [CN V] or tongue [CN XII])? Conditions such as an acoustic neuroma and Ramsay–Hunt syndrome can affect the cranial nerves.

EXAMINATION

Examination of the ear for hearing loss should include the following:

- Inspection for pinna symmetry and deformity (e.g. swelling), presence of scars and hearing aids
- Palpate the tragus and mastoid for tenderness
- Using an otoscope, examine the external auditory canal looking for evidence of wax, erythema, discharge, vesicles or masses. Examine the tympanic membrane looking for the light reflex. Look for evidence of perforation, retraction (Eustachian tube dysfunction) or bulging (otitis media). Look in the attic for the presence of a cholesteatoma
- Perform Rinne's and Weber's test (using a short 512-Hz tuning fork)
  - Rinne's test: With the tuning fork vibrating, place it on the patient's mastoid and ask the patient to tell you when they can no longer hear it. Then move the tuning fork in front of the ear (2 cm away from the meatus). If they can still hear it, this means the test is positive (normal) and that air conduction is better than bone conduction (AC>BC)
  - Weber's test: With the tuning fork vibrating, place it on the patient's forehead and ask them where they can hear it loudest: centrally, left or right. Normally, the result is centrally

Interpretations of Rinne's and Weber's

Positive (normal) Rinne's bilaterally and Weber's central = Normal.

Abnormal Rinne's on the right and Weber's lateralising to the right = Conductive hearing loss on the right.

Abnormal Rinne's on the right and Weber's lateralising to the left = Sensorineural hearing loss on the right.

INVESTIGATIONS

Bedside: Rinne's and Weber's test, otoscopy, audiometry, PTA, tympanometry

Imaging: MRI head

MANAGEMENT

Referral to ENT should be made in any patient with:

- Conductive deafness of unknown cause
- Sudden deafness if no wax is visible on examination
- Asymmetrical deafness (to exclude more sinister causes of deafness like acoustic neuroma/cholesteatoma)

Management of hearing loss will depend on the cause – management of common causes of hearing loss is listed here.

Presbyacusis

Once diagnosis is confirmed by audiometry, then patients should be referred for a hearing aid if appropriate.

Wax

Patients should be educated about wax and discouraged from using objects to clean the ear (e.g. cotton buds).

Ear syringing is indicated if the wax is causing symptoms of deafness or pain. Avoid syringing if perforation or chronic middle ear disease. If syringing is contraindicated or unsuccessful, refer to ENT for removal under direct vision (microsuction).

Otitis media

Look for complications of otitis media (meningitis, mastoiditis or facial nerve paralysis) and admit if present.

Admit patients who are systemically unwell or are children <3 months old or 3–6 months with a fever >39°C.

Otherwise: Treat pain and fever with paracetamol/NSAIDs. Most people do not need antibiotics but consider if systemically unwell, >4 days of non-improving symptoms, perforation, bilateral otitis media. If an adult goes on to develop otitis media with effusion (OME) then refer them to ENT to exclude a nasopharyngeal cancer.

Otosclerosis

Referral to ENT may be required for assessment to replace the stapes with an implant or bone-anchored hearing aid.

Acoustic neuroma

Referral to ENT for investigations.

Any patient with unilateral or asymmetrical sensorineural hearing loss/tinnitus and balance problems should be referred urgently to ENT!

Menière's disease

See Section 15.1 for the management of Menière's disease.

Table 15.2.1 Causes of hearing loss

Conductive	Sensorineural
Wax	Presbyacusis
Acute otitis media	Noise-induced hearing loss (NIHL)
Otosclerosis	Menière's disease
Barotrauma	Acoustic neuroma
Tympanic membrane injury	Drug-induced (e.g. aminoglycosides, loop diuretics)
Cholesteatoma	Ramsay–Hunt syndrome
	Congenital causes (e.g. Alport's syndrome)

EAR, NOSE AND THROAT: QUESTIONS

15.1 VERTIGO

1. What is the most commonly diagnosed cause of vertigo?

2. What is the difference between acute vestibular neuronitis and acute labyrinthitis?

3. What investigation needs to be performed before the diagnosis of Menière's disease and why?

4. A 76-year-old woman is diagnosed with Menière's disease. What treatment options are available to her?

5. What treatment options are available for symptomatic relief of acute vestibular neuronitis and labyrinthitis?

15.2 HEARING LOSS

1. Classify the following causes of hearing loss by whether they predominantly cause:
   a. Conductive hearing loss

   b. Sensorineural hearing loss
      i. Acoustic neuroma
      ii. Otosclerosis
      iii. Wax
      iv. Presbyacusis
      v. Ramsay–Hunt syndrome
      vi. Noise-induced hearing loss
      vii. Otitis media
      viii. Menière's disease

2. What red flag features should you look for when a patient presents with acute otitis media?

3. In which scenarios when a patient presents with hearing loss should you always refer to ENT?

4. Which medications can lead to a sensorineural hearing loss?

CHAPTER **16**

Answers

Chapter 1: CARDIOLOGY

1.1 ACUTE CORONARY SYNDROME

1. What are the risk factors for an acute coronary syndrome?

   Risk factors for ACS can be divided into modifiable and non-modifiable:

   Modifiable risk factors: Hypertension, smoking, ↑ cholesterol, diabetes, obesity, sedentary lifestyle.

   Non-modifiable risk factors: Family history, ↑ age, sex (M > F).

2. Outline the initial prehospital management for an acute coronary syndrome.

   Initial management for ACS can be remembered by the mnemonic **M²ONA**:

   Morphine, **M**etoclopramide, **O**xygen (if <94%), **N**itrates (only if ongoing pain), **A**spirin 300 mg.

3. What are the complications of a myocardial infarction?

   Complications post-MI include **ischaemic** complications (angina, re-infarction), **mechanical** complications (heart failure, mitral valve dysfunction, ventricular wall rupture), **arrhythmic** complications (heart block, ventricular tachycardia/fibrillation), **embolic** complications (lodging into the peripheral circulation/carotid territory) and **inflammatory** complications (early pericarditis and Dressler syndrome).

1.2 HEART FAILURE

1. Name three signs of both left-sided and right-sided heart failure that you may elicit on examination.

   Signs of left-sided heart failure: Fine bibasal crepitations, displaced apex beat, gallop rhythm, JVP may be elevated due to back pressure through lungs.

   Signs of right-sided heart failure: ↑ JVP, peripheral oedema, hepatomegaly, ascites, reduced air entry, dull percussion note.

2. How do you manage a patient presenting with acute pulmonary oedema?

   You would manage them with an ABCDE approach. The mnemonic used in this book is **IPODMAN**:

   Intravenous access, **P**osition the patient (upright), **O**xygen (high-flow), **D**iuretic (IV furosemide), **M**orphine, **A**ntiemetic, **N**itrates. CPAP can also be used to improve oxygenation.

3. Which drugs have been shown to improve mortality in patients with chronic heart failure?

ACE inhibitors, beta-blockers, spironolactone, hydralazine with nitrates; more recently ivabradine in tachycardic patients and sacubitril/valsartan.

1.3 HYPERTENSION

1. What conservative and medical treatments would you consider in the management of a 56-year-old Caucasian woman with stage 2 hypertension?

   Conservative: Education about the condition, lifestyle advice (diet/exercise/smoking/alcohol), check for complications.

   Medical: Initial step is the introduction of a calcium channel blocker.

2. Which investigations would you perform to look for evidence of end-organ damage in a hypertensive patient?

   Urinalysis/U&Es for kidney damage, ophthalmoscopy for retinopathy, ECG for evidence of LVH.

1.4 VALVULAR HEART DISEASE

1. What features may you find on cardiovascular examination in a patient with aortic stenosis?

   Ejection systolic murmur (heard loudest over the second R intercostal space and radiates to the carotids), narrow pulse pressure, left ventricular hypertrophy.

2. What features may you find on cardiovascular examination in a patient with mitral regurgitation?

   Pan-systolic murmur to be heard at the apex of the heart radiating to the axilla.

   Patients may be in AF and have a displaced thrusting apex (signs of fluid overload).

   Soft S1, LVF (S3, pulmonary oedema), loud P2 and right ventricular heave (pulmonary hypertension).

3. How would a patient with symptomatic aortic stenosis present in comparison to a patient with symptomatic mitral regurgitation?

   Patients with aortic stenosis may present with **SAD** (exertional **S**yncope, **A**ngina and **D**yspnoea).

   Patients with mitral regurgitation may present with dyspnoea, palpitations and fluid overload.

1.5 INFECTIVE ENDOCARDITIS

1. Which organisms most commonly cause infective endocarditis?

   Staphylococcus aureus, Streptococcus viridans, Staphylococcus epidermidis.

2. What signs may you elicit on examination in patients with infective endocarditis?

There are **nine** signs of infective endocarditis that may be elicited on examination:

Fever, clubbing, splinter haemorrhages, Osler nodes, Janeway lesions, Roth spots, murmur, splenomegaly, haematuria.

3. Outline the two major Duke criteria for diagnosis of infective endocarditis.

    Positive blood cultures (typical organisms on two separate occasions or persistent bacteraemia from two blood cultures taken >12 hours apart).

    Endocardium involvement (positive echocardiogram showing a vegetation or abscess or a new valvular regurgitation or direct histological or microbiological confirmation from a pathological specimen).

1.6 ATRIAL FIBRILLATION

1. Name three causes of atrial fibrillation.

    Any three from: (see table below)

2. What ECG features are suggestive of atrial fibrillation?

    An irregularly irregular rhythm with absence of p waves.

3. What are the initial options available to rate control a patient with atrial fibrillation, providing no contraindications?

    Initial options include either a beta-blocker or rate-limiting calcium channel blocker.

Cardiac	Respiratory	Endocrine	Other
Hypertension	Pneumonia	Thyrotoxicosis	Infection
IHD (from muscle damage)	PE	Diabetes mellitus	Drugs (thyroxine)
Valvular disease (e.g. mitral stenosis)	Pleural effusion		Alcohol
Cardiomyopathy	Lung cancer		Electrolyte disturbance

CHAPTER 2: RESPIRATORY

2.1 ASTHMA

1. What are the risk factors for the development of asthma?

   Risk factors for the development of asthma include history (personal or family) of atopy, allergen exposure, occupation (e.g. chemical irritants in the workplace [e.g. flour dust/isocyanates from paint]), outdoor cold air/exercise/extreme emotional arousal and medications (such as NSAIDs, aspirin, beta-blockers).

2. Which tests are performed for a new diagnosis of asthma?

   The diagnostic testing for asthma in adults includes having a spirometry with a bronchodilator reversibility test and an FeNO test.

3. Which medications are used in an acute exacerbation of asthma?

   Medications used in an acute exacerbation of asthma include: **SONS**: Steroids, Oxygen, Nebulisers (salbutamol/ipratropium bromide), Magnesium Sulphate.

2.2 CHRONIC OBSTRUCTIVE PULMONARY DISEASE

1. What is the greatest aetiological factor for the development of COPD?

   Smoking is by far the biggest aetiological factor for the development of COPD.

2. Which organisms commonly cause an infective exacerbation of COPD?

   Infective exacerbations are most commonly due to the bacterial organisms *Haemophilus influenzae* and *Streptococcus pneumoniae*.

3. What are the management options for COPD?

   Conservative management options include stopping smoking, education about the condition, vaccinations and involving the multidisciplinary team.

   Medical management options include using a short-acting beta-2-agonist (SABA) or short-acting muscarinic antagonist (SAMA) initially followed by (if asthmatic features present) either a long-acting beta-2-agonist (LABA) with an inhaled corticosteroid (ICS) or (if no asthmatic features or steroid responsiveness) a LABA + LAMA. Other options include mucolytics, theophylline, roflumilast and long-term oxygen therapy (LTOT).

2.3 PNEUMONIA

1. Which organisms commonly cause a community-acquired pneumonia?

   The two most common organisms causing CAP are *Streptococcus pneumoniae* and *Haemophilus influenzae*.

2. What makes up the CURB-65 score for the management of community-acquired pneumonia?

   The CURB-65 score is made up of: **C**onfusion, **U**rea, **R**espiratory rate, **B**lood pressure, age ≥**65** years.

2.4 INTERSTITIAL LUNG DISEASE

1. What are the causes of interstitial lung disease?

   Causes of ILD include:

   - Infection (e.g. TB, atypical pneumonia)
   - Inhaled irritants (e.g. inorganic irritants such as in silicosis, asbestosis, berylliosis or organic irritants causing extrinsic allergic alveolitis)
   - Idiopathic (e.g. IPF, sarcoidosis, antisynthetase syndrome)
   - Malignancy (e.g. lymphangitis carcinomatosa)
   - Connective tissue disease (e.g. SLE, RA, dermatomyositis, polymyositis, systemic sclerosis)
   - Drugs (e.g. nitrofurantoin, methotrexate, amiodarone, sulfasalazine, simvastatin)

2. What is cor pulmonale and what are the ECG findings?

   Cor pulmonale refers to enlargement and failure of the right side of the heart as a result of increased vascular resistance in the lungs. ECG findings may include right axis deviation, p pulmonale or right ventricular hypertrophy.

3. Which medications can be used to treat idiopathic pulmonary fibrosis?

   Medications include oxygen, pirfenidone and nintedanib.

2.5 LUNG CANCER

1. What are the presenting features of lung cancer?

   Patients with lung cancer may present with respiratory symptoms (e.g. cough, haemoptysis, shortness of breath), chest pain, recurrent infections, systemic symptoms (fatigue, weight loss) or symptoms from a paraneoplastic syndrome or metastases.

2. What is the most common type of lung cancer?

   Non-small cell lung cancer (NSCLC) is the most common type of lung cancer.

3. What are the paraneoplastic syndromes that can occur with lung cancer?

Paraneoplastic syndromes that may occur with lung cancer include:

- Hypercalcaemia (due to ↑ PTHrP secretion in squamous cell lung cancer)

- SIADH (due to ↑ ADH secretion in a small-cell lung cancer)

- Cushing syndrome (due to ↑ ACTH secretion in a small-cell lung cancer)

- Lambert–Eaton syndrome (due to antibodies to voltage gated calcium channels in small-cell lung cancer)

CHAPTER 3: GASTROENTEROLOGY

3.1 CROHN'S DISEASE

1. Which part of the gastrointestinal tract does Crohn's disease affect?

   Crohn's disease can affect anywhere along the gastrointestinal tract – from mouth to anus. It most commonly affects the terminal ileum. Crohn's disease causes transmural inflammation of the gastrointestinal tract, meaning that all layers of the gastrointestinal wall are affected.

2. Which vitamin and nutrient deficiencies should be screened for in patients with Crohn's disease?

   Patients should be screened for serum ferritin, vitamin B_{12}, folate, calcium and vitamin D to check for deficiency.

3. What are the extra-intestinal features of inflammatory bowel disease?

   The extra-intestinal features of inflammatory bowel disease include **C-3P-O**: **C**lubbing, e**P**iscleritis, **P**yoderma gangrenosum/erythema nodosum, **P**ainful joints (arthritis) and **O**steoporosis.

3.2 ULCERATIVE COLITIS

1. Which part of the gastrointestinal tract does ulcerative colitis affect?

   Ulcerative colitis affects the **large bowel**, and the inflammatory process starts in the rectum before spreading proximally. It does not extend beyond the ileocaecal valve. UC only affects the mucosa of the GI tract.

2. What are the features of a severe flare of ulcerative colitis?

   Features of a severe flare include:
   - More than six liquid stools/day
   - Severe rectal bleeding
   - Pyrexia >37.8, ↑ WCC
   - Signs of shock (↑ pulse, ↓ blood pressure)
   - ↑ ESR (>30), ↓ Hb (<10.5)

3.3 COELIAC DISEASE

1. What are the pathological changes in the small bowel in coeliac disease?

   There is villous atrophy and crypt hyperplasia of the small intestine due to repeated gluten exposure in a sensitive individual.

2. What clinical signs may you elicit in a patient with coeliac disease?

   Patients may be underweight due to malabsorption, and have signs of aphthous ulceration, angular stomatitis (iron deficiency), dermatitis herpetiformis (IgA deposition in the skin) and have polyneuropathy secondary to folate/B_{12} deficiency.

3. What are the first-line investigations for the diagnosis of coeliac disease?

   Immunoglobulin A (IgA) tissue transglutaminase antibody (tTGA) and total IgA are first-line investigations.

3.4 LIVER FAILURE

1. Name three causes of acute liver failure.

   Any three from: Infection (e.g. hepatitis/Weil's disease), drugs (e.g. paracetamol overdose), vascular causes (Budd–Chiari), infiltration (e.g. Wilson's) and acute-on-chronic causes such as alcohol binging and GI bleeding.

2. What are the features of liver decompensation?

   Features include hepatic encephalopathy (↑ ammonia), bleeding (↓ clotting) and ascites (↓ albumin).

3. What are the signs of liver failure that may be elicited on examination?

   Signs of liver failure include jaundice, gynaecomastia, spider naevi (found in distribution of IVC), bruising.

   Hand signs such as clubbing, white nails (low albumin), Dupuytren's contracture, palmar erythema, asterixis.

   Abdominal signs such as skin telangiectasia, oedema, ascites, caput medusa, hypogonadism.

   Abdominal findings such as hepatomegaly (not in cirrhosis), splenomegaly (from portal hypertension).

3.5 JAUNDICE

1. What are the causes of prehepatic jaundice and what will the LFTs likely show?

   Causes of prehepatic jaundice include haemolytic anaemias, medications (e.g. antimalarials) and glucuronyl transferase deficiencies (e.g. Gilbert's syndrome or Crigler–Najjar syndrome). LFTs will show a raised bilirubin.

2. What are the causes of intrahepatic jaundice and what will the LFTs likely show?

   Causes of intrahepatic jaundice include hepatitis, alcoholic liver disease, hepatocellular carcinoma, right-sided heart failure, Budd–Chiari syndrome, drugs (e.g. paracetamol overdose) and infiltrative diseases (e.g. Wilson's, haemochromatosis). LFTs will show a raised bilirubin and ALT/AST (much higher than GGT or ALP).

3. What are the causes of posthepatic jaundice and what will the LFTs likely show?

Causes of posthepatic jaundice include gall-stones, pancreatitis, pancreatic cancer, cholangiocarcinoma, drugs (e.g. co-amoxiclav) and autoimmune conditions (e.g. PBC, PSC). LFTs will show a raised bilirubin and ALP/GGT (much higher than ALT and AST).

3.6 UPPER GASTROINTESTINAL BLEED

1. Name three causes of upper gastrointestinal bleeding

   Any from: Peptic ulcer disease, oesophageal varices, Mallory–Weiss tear, inflammation (gastritis/oesophagitis), and malignancy (gastric/oesophageal). Other causes include arterio-venous malformations, drugs (e.g. warfarin), bleeding disorders and hereditary haemorrhagic telangiectasia (HHT).

2. What are the scoring systems used when a patient presents with an upper gastrointestinal bleed?

   The Glasgow–Blatchford score (preendoscopy) to identify patients who will need endoscopic management and the Rockall score (postendoscopy) to identify patients at a high risk of adverse outcomes following a bleed.

3. Which medications are often given to patients with oesophageal varices prior to their endoscopy?

   Patients with bleeding oesophageal varices are often given prophylactic antibiotics and terlipressin, an ADH analogue that reduces portal system pressure, prior to endoscopy.

CHAPTER 4: ENDOCRINOLOGY

4.1 TYPE 2 DIABETES MELLITUS

1. Name three risk factors for the development of type 2 diabetes mellitus.

   Any three from:

   Genetic risk factors (increased risk if a first-degree relative has the condition)

   Environmental risk factors: Obesity, lack of physical activity, a history of gestational diabetes and medications (e.g. corticosteroids, atypical antipsychotics) and causes of secondary diabetes (e.g. chronic pancreatitis).

2. What are the macrovascular and microvascular complications of type 2 diabetes mellitus?

   Macrovascular complications include peripheral vascular disease, ischaemic heart disease and cerebrovascular disease. Microvascular complications include diabetic retinopathy, nephropathy and neuropathy.

3. How can type 2 diabetes mellitus be diagnosed?

   Type 2 diabetes mellitus can be diagnosed from a single raised blood glucose reading if the patient is symptomatic (either fasting glucose ≥ 7.0 mmol/L or random glucose ≥ 11.1 mmol/L) or two high readings if the patient is asymptomatic. HbA1c $\geq 6.5\%$ (48 mmol/mol) is also diagnostic.

4. What are the mechanisms of action of the drugs metformin, gliclazide and dapagliflozin?

   Metformin is a biguanide that reduces the rate of gluconeogenesis and increases insulin sensitivity.

   Gliclazide is a sulphonylurea that promotes insulin secretion from pancreatic beta cells.

   Dapagliflozin is a sodium–glucose transport protein 2 inhibitor that prevents glucose reabsorption in the kidney.

4.2 HYPOTHYROIDISM

1. What signs may be elicited on examination in a patient with hypothyroidism?

   Signs include increased body weight, dry skin, thin hair, cold hands, bradycardia, myxoedema, periorbital oedema, goitre, slow-relaxing biceps reflex and proximal myopathy.

2. Name three causes of hypothyroidism.

   Any three from primary atrophic hypothyroidism, Hashimoto's thyroiditis, iodine deficiency, medications (e.g. amiodarone), subacute thyroiditis and Reidel's thyroiditis.

3. Which autoimmune conditions are associated with autoimmune hypothyroidism?

   Type 1 diabetes mellitus, vitiligo, coeliac disease, pernicious anaemia.

4.3 HYPERTHYROIDISM

1. Which antibodies may be present in Graves' disease?

   TSH-receptor antibodies.

2. What are the medical management options for hyperthyroidism?

   Symptomatic treatment (beta-blocker e.g. propranolol).

   Anti-thyroid regimes: Titration with carbimazole or block and replace with carbimazole and levothyroxine.

3. What are the complications of hyperthyroidism?

   Complications include cardiovascular problems (heart failure, AF), osteoporosis and ophthalmopathy.

4.4 CUSHING'S SYNDROME

1. What are the ACTH-dependent causes of Cushing's syndrome?

   ACTH-dependent causes of Cushing's syndrome include Cushing's disease (pituitary adenoma) and ectopic secretion (e.g. from a small-cell lung cancer).

2. What are the ACTH-independent causes of Cushing's syndrome?

   ACTH-independent causes of Cushing's syndrome include iatrogenic (e.g. corticosteroids), adrenal adenoma and adrenal carcinoma.

3. What tests can be performed to confirm the presence of Cushing's syndrome?

   Confirmation tests include the overnight dexamethasone suppression tests and 24-hour urinary free cortisol collection.

4.5 ADRENAL GLAND DISORDERS

1. What are the layers of the adrenal cortex and what do they produce?

   Remember **GFR**:

   - **G**lomerulosa (produces aldosterone).
   - **F**asciculata (produces cortisol).
   - **R**eticularis (produces precursor androgens, e.g. DHEA)

2. What is the definitive diagnostic test for Addison's disease?

   Short Synacthen test.

3. What are the electrolyte abnormalities seen in primary hyperaldosteronism?

   Hypernatraemia and hypokalaemia. The loss of H^+ in the kidneys leads to a metabolic alkalosis.

CHAPTER 5: RHEUMATOLOGY

5.1 RHEUMATOID ARTHRITIS

1. Name three extra-articular manifestations of rheumatoid arthritis.

   Any three from:

   - **C**ardiac involvement: Pericarditis, endocarditis, ischaemic heart disease.
   - **R**espiratory involvement: Pleural effusions, interstitial lung disease, Caplan syndrome.
   - **O**cular involvement: Keratoconjunctivitis sicca, episcleritis, scleritis.
   - **C**irculation: Anaemia of chronic disease, vasculitis, amyloidosis, Felty's syndrome.
   - **S**oft-tissue: Rheumatoid nodules, carpal tunnel syndrome, atlanto-axial subluxation, palmar erythema, osteoporosis, subaxial subluxation.
   - Depression can also be considered an extra-articular manifestation.

2. What medications can be used in the treatment of rheumatoid arthritis?

   Medications include analgesics (e.g. paracetamol, NSAIDs, COX-inhibitors), corticosteroids, DMARD therapies (such as methotrexate, hydroxychloroquine, leflunomide, sulfasalazine), biologics (such as etanercept, rituximab) and JAK2 inhibitors (such as baricitinib).

3. What are the side effects of methotrexate?

   Side effects of methotrexate include neutropenia, renal impairment, GI disturbance, pneumonitis, pulmonary fibrosis and deranged LFTs (including cirrhosis).

5.2 SERONEGATIVE SPONDYLOARTHROPATHIES

1. What features do the seronegative spondyloarthropathies share?

   Seronegative spondyloarthropathies:

   - Have a negative rheumatoid factor
   - Are associated with HLA-B27
   - Iritis
   - Generally affect the spine and peripheral joints

Psoriatic arthritis

1. What is the most common form of psoriatic arthritis?

The most common type of psoriatic arthritis is a peripheral symmetrical polyarthritis (similar to RA).

2. What are the treatment options for psoriatic arthritis?

   Treatment options include simple analgesia and NSAIDs for joint pain; DMARDs, anti-TNFs and biologics can now be utilised to help manage both the arthralgia and skin disease. Specific medications include apremilast, secukinumab and ixekizumab.

Ankylosing spondylitis

1. What is the clinical test for reduced lumbar flexion in ankylosing spondylitis?

   Schober's test

2. What are the extra-articular manifestations of ankylosing spondylitis?

   The 5 **A**s: **A**nterior uveitis, **A**ortic incompetence, **A**myloidosis, **A**pical lung fibrosis, **A**V block.

Reactive arthritis

1. What are the extra-articular signs and symptoms of reactive arthritis?

   Extra-articular signs and symptoms of reactive arthritis include urethritis, conjunctivitis, circinate balanitis and keratoderma blennorrhagica.

2. What is the classic triad of symptoms in reactive arthritis?

   The triad consists of arthralgia, conjunctivitis and urethritis.

5.3 SYSTEMIC LUPUS ERYTHEMATOSUS

1. Name three organs SLE can affect and the manifestations from its involvement.

   Any three from:

   - Joints: Peripheral small joint arthritis
   - Skin: Malar (butterfly) rash, photosensitive rash, discoid lupus, livedo reticularis, Raynaud's phenomenon, alopecia
   - Nervous system: Seizures/psychosis, mood disorder and anxiety can occur, migraine
   - Respiratory: Pleuritic, fibrosing alveolitis
   - Kidneys: Lupus nephritis
   - Cardiovascular: Pericarditis, myocarditis, pericardial effusions, vasculitis, endocarditis
   - Gastroenterology: Oral ulcers

- Haematology: Haemolytic anaemia, lympho-penia, thrombocytopenia, antiphospholipid syndrome

2. Which medications can cause drug-induced lupus?

   Drugs include hydralazine, procainamide, penicil-lamine and isoniazid.

3. What management options are available for treating SLE?

   Management options include:

   - Conservative options: Avoid triggers, assess risk for cardiovascular disease and osteoporosis.
   - Use of topical steroids and high-factor sunblock.
   - NSAIDs for joint pain.
   - DMARD therapy (such as hydroxychloro-quine). Some biologics can be used.

5.4 GOUT

1. Name three risk factors for the development of gout.

   Any three from:

   - Hyperuricaemia (either from impaired renal excretion of urate or secondary causes such as hypertension)
   - Increasing age
   - Male gender
   - Menopausal women
   - Chronic kidney disease
   - Obesity and metabolic syndrome
   - Diet (high-purine diet, e.g. beer)
   - Drugs (diuretics)

2. How should an acute attack of gout be managed and what medications can be used?

   Patients should rest the affected joint and modify lifestyle issues that predispose to a flare of acute gout. Patients should have pharmacological man-agement in the form of an NSAID (with a co-pre-scribed PPI) or oral colchicine. If patients cannot tolerate NSAIDs or colchicine, corticosteroids (oral/IM) can be considered.

   Urate-lowering therapies (such as allopurinol or febuxostat) should not be initiated or stopped during an acute attack of gout.

3. How do the crystals of gout differ from those that cause pseudogout?

   The crystals seen following arthrocentesis in gout are negatively birefringent needle-shaped crystals. In pseudogout, they are positively bire-fringent rhomboid-shaped crystals.

5.5 OSTEOPOROSIS

1. Name three risk factors for osteoporosis.

   Any three from:

   - **S**teroid use
   - **H**yperthyroidism/**H**yperparathyroidism
   - **A**lcohol and tobacco use
   - **T**hin (BMI <18.5)
   - **T**estosterone ↓
   - **E**arly menopause
   - **R**enal or liver failure
   - **E**rosive bone disease (e.g. myeloma, RA)
   - **D**ietary Ca^{2+} ↓/**D**iabetes

2. Other than osteoporosis, what can cause a fragil-ity fracture?

   Non-osteoporotic causes of a fragility fracture include:

   - Metastatic bone disease
   - Multiple myeloma
   - Osteomalacia
   - Paget's disease of bone

3. What pharmacological therapies can be used to treat osteoporosis?

   Pharmacological options for treating osteoporosis include bisphosphonates (e.g. alendronate), ral-oxifene, denosumab, teriparatide, vitamin D and calcium supplementation.

CHAPTER 6: NEUROLOGY

6.1 STROKE/TIA

1. Name three risk factors for an ischaemic stroke.

   Any three from:
   - Lifestyle factors (modifiable): Smoking, alcohol/drug misuse, physical inactivity and poor diet
   - Previous cardiovascular disease: Hypertension, atrial fibrillation, carotid artery disease, infective endocarditis, valvular heart disease, congestive cardiac failure
   - Other factors: Age, hyperlipidaemia, DM, CKD, COCP, OSA, hypercoagulable disorders

2. Within what time frame of stroke symptoms should thrombolysis be given in an ischaemic stroke, provided there are no contraindications?

   4.5 hours

6.2 PARKINSON'S DISEASE

1. Name three causes of parkinsonism.
   - Idiopathic Parkinson's disease
   - Cerebral infarctions
   - Drug-induced (prochlorperazine, metoclopramide)
   - Infiltrative diseases (Wilson's)
   - Parkinson's-plus syndromes (progressive nuclear palsy [PSP], multiple system atrophy [MSA], corticobasal degeneration [CBD], Lewy-body dementia)

2. Name three features of parkinsonism.

   Any three from: Tremor, rigidity, akinesia, postural instability.

6.3 EPILEPSY

Vanessa is a 27-year-old woman who suffers with generalised tonic–clonic seizures that are managed with sodium valproate.

1. Name two side effects of sodium valproate.

   Any two from: Nausea, increased appetite and weight gain, alopecia (regrowth may be curly), ataxia, tremor, hepatitis, pancreatitis, thrombocytopenia, teratogenicity.

2. Vanessa is interested in driving again. How long does she need to be seizure-free before being able to drive?

   12 months.

6.4 MULTIPLE SCLEROSIS

1. What are the different patterns of multiple sclerosis?

   Relapsing–remitting, secondary progressive, primary progressive.

2. What are the complications of multiple sclerosis?

   Complications include fatigue, spasticity, decreased mobility, depression, pain, bladder and bowel problems and sexual dysfunction.

6.5 MIGRAINE/HEADACHE

1. What features in a headache history support a diagnosis of migraine?

   Unilateral nature, pulsatile, lasting hours to days, associated with gastrointestinal symptoms, photophobia and phonophobia, need to rest, transient focal neurological disturbance and aura.

2. What medication can be offered to patients as prophylaxis for migraine attacks?

   Options include propranolol and topiramate.

6.6 NEUROPATHIES

1. Guillain–Barré syndrome classically has what features on examination?

   Weakness in all four limbs (ascending), mild sensory signs, areflexia, cranial nerve involvement.

2. What are the causes of carpal tunnel syndrome?

   MEDIAN TRAP: **M**yxoedema, o**E**dema, **D**iabetes, **I**diopathic, **A**cromegaly, **N**eoplasm, **T**rauma, **R**heumatoid arthritis, **A**myloidosis, **P**regnancy.

6.7 CEREBELLAR SYNDROME

1. Name three signs of cerebellar syndrome that can be elicited on examination.

   Any three from **DANISH**: **D**ysdiadochokinesis, **A**taxia, **N**ystagmus, **I**ntention tremor, **S**lurred/staccato speech, **H**ypotonia.

2. Name three causes of cerebellar syndrome.

   Demyelination (e.g. MS)
   - Alcohol
   - Stroke
   - Space-occupying lesion
   - Inherited (Wilson's, Friedrich's ataxia)
   - Drugs (antiepileptics)
   - Multiple system atrophy

CHAPTER 7: RENAL AND ELECTROLYTES

7.1 ACUTE KIDNEY INJURY

1. Name three causes of acute kidney injury.

    Prerenal causes: Hypovolaemia (e.g. secondary to sepsis), reduced cardiac output.

    Renal causes: Nephrotoxic drugs, vasculitis, glomerulonephritis, acute tubular necrosis, rhabdomyosis, myeloma, interstitial nephritis.

    Postrenal causes: Renal stones, blocked catheter, pelvic mass, benign prostatic hypertrophy, prostate cancer, cervical cancer, retroperitoneal fibrosis.

2. Name two signs of acute renal failure you may see on examination.

    *   Reduced urine output
    *   Pulmonary and peripheral oedema
    *   Arrhythmias (due to ↑ K^+)
    *   Features of uraemia (e.g. pericarditis or encephalopathy)

3. Name the three changes you may see in the U&Es for a patient in an acute kidney injury.

    *   Raised urea
    *   Raised creatinine
    *   Raised potassium (hyperkalaemia)

7.2 CHRONIC KIDNEY DISEASE

1. Name three causes of chronic kidney disease.

    DR CABG: **D**iabetes/**D**rugs, **R**enal infection, **C**ongenital (polycystic kidney disease), **A**utoimmune (SLE/vasculitis), **B**lood pressure (hypertension), **G**lomerulonephritis.

2. An eGFR of 25 corresponds to which stage of chronic kidney disease?

    Stage 4.

3. Name three medical treatments used in the management of chronic kidney disease.

    *   Antihypertensives (e.g. ACE inhibitor/ARB)
    *   Antiplatelets (e.g. aspirin)
    *   Antilipids (e.g. atorvastatin)
    *   Binders (phosphate)
    *   Bicarbonate (oral)
    *   Calcium supplementation
    *   EPO stimulators for anaemia (if suitable)

ELECTROLYTE IMBALANCES

1. Name three drugs associated with hyponatraemia.

    SSRIs, diuretics (e.g. loop diuretics), NSAIDs, TCAs, carbamazepine, antipsychotics.

2. What are the ECG changes associated with hyperkalaemia?

    *   Small/absent p waves
    *   Broad and wide QRS
    *   Tall tented T waves

3. What are the symptoms of hypercalcaemia?

    Bones (bone pain), stones (renal calculi), groans (abdominal pain, tiredness/weakness), thrones (polydipsia, constipation), psychic moans (confusion).

CHAPTER 8: HAEMATOLOGY

8.1 ANAEMIA

1. How are anaemias classified?

   Anaemias are classified by size of the red blood cell – the mean cell volume (MCV). The three broad categories of anaemia are microcytic, normocytic and macrocytic.

2. What can cause a microcytic anaemia?

   The most common cause of a microcytic anaemia is iron deficiency anaemia (IDA). Thalassaemia can also cause a microcytic anaemia.

3. What is the most common cause of iron deficiency anaemia in men and postmenopausal women?

   Blood loss from the gastrointestinal tract.

4. What can cause a macrocytic anaemia?

   The differential for a macrocytic anaemia includes vitamin B_{12} deficiency, folate deficiency, haemolytic anaemias, hypothyroidism, liver disease, drugs and myelodysplasia.

5. What blood results would be suggestive of a haemolytic anaemia?

   A normocytic or macrocytic anaemia

   A raised unconjugated bilirubin and LDH

   A blood film may also show spherocytes (if immune-mediated or hereditary spherocytosis)

8.2 HAEMATOLOGICAL MALIGNANCIES

1. How are leukaemias classified?

   Leukaemias are classified into the cell line from which they originate (lymphocyte vs. myeloid) and whether they occur acutely or chronically. This gives four broad groups of leukaemias:

   - Acute lymphoblastic leukaemia (ALL)
   - Chronic lymphocytic leukaemia (CLL)
   - Acute myeloid leukaemia (AML)
   - Chronic myeloid leukaemia (CML)

2. The Philadelphia chromosome is a translocation between which two chromosomes?

   The Philadelphia chromosome is a translocation between chromosomes 9 and 22.

3. Which cell is classically found in affected lymph nodes of patients with Hodgkin's lymphoma?

   The Reed–Sternberg cell.

4. Name the four myeloproliferative disorders.

   (1) Polycythaemia rubra vera, (2) essential thrombocytosis, (3) myelofibrosis and (4) CML.

5. Multiple myeloma is a proliferation of which immune cell?

   Multiple myeloma occurs as a result of proliferation of abnormal plasma cells.

CHAPTER 9: INFECTIOUS DISEASES

9.1 HEPATITIS

1. Name three causes of hepatitis.

   Any three from: Viral hepatitis (e.g. hepatitis A–E, EBV, CMV), autoimmune causes (e.g. auto-immune hepatitis, PBC, PSC), infiltrative causes (e.g. sarcoidosis, Wilson's, haemochromatosis), metabolic causes (e.g. NAFLD, alcoholic-liver disease, alpa-1-antitrypsin deficiency) and drugs (e.g. methotrexate, amiodarone, isoniazid).

2. Which viral hepatitis can lead to chronic liver failure?

   Hepatitis B (10%–15%) and hepatitis C (50%–80%).

3. What would the immunological profile of a patient who has a resolved hepatitis B infection look like?

   Negative HBsAg, positive anti-HBc, positive anti-HBs.

9.2 MENINGITIS

1. What features of CSF analysis are suggestive of bacterial meningitis?

   Cloudy CSF, low glucose, high protein, high poly-morphs.

2. A 22-year-old man presents with symptoms of meningitis. CSF isolates a gram-negative diplo-coccus. What is the causative organism?

   Neisseria meningitidis.

9.3 HIV

1. What are the symptoms of acute retroviral syndrome?

   Acute retroviral syndrome occurs 2–6 weeks after exposure and causes symptoms such as malaise, fever, sore throat, lymphadenopathy, diarrhoea, arthralgia, aphthous ulceration and a maculopapular rash.

2. Which tests are considered first-line to diagnose HIV? What are the 'window periods'?

   The combined HIV antibody and p24 antigen tests are considered first-line to diagnose HIV. These fourth-generation tests have a window period of 4 weeks.

3. Name three complications of HIV infection.

   Any three from:
   - Acute retroviral syndrome
   - Persistent generalised lymphadenopathy
   - Progression to AIDS
   - Recurrent infections (e.g. pneumonia)

   - Respiratory complications, e.g. *Pneumocystis jirovecii* pneumonia, *Cryptococcus*, TB
   - Neurological complications, e.g. cerebral toxoplasmosis, cryptococcal meningitis, primary CNS
   - Lymphoma, encephalitis (CMV/HIV), progressive multifocal leukoencephalopathy (PML), AIDS dementia complex
   - Gastrointestinal, e.g. candidiasis, diarrhoea (e.g. cryptosporidium)
   - Skin, e.g. Kaposi's sarcoma
   - Eye, e.g. CMV retinitis
   - Cancer, e.g. non-Hodgkin's lymphoma, Burkitt's lymphoma
   - Psychological, e.g. depression

4. How long post-exposure can PEPSE medications be given?

   PEPSE can be given up to 72 hours after exposure. It is ideally given within the first 24 hours.

5. Which classes of medications are given to patients with a new diagnosis of HIV?

   Patients with a new diagnosis of HIV are recommended to be treated with two nucleoside reverse transcriptase inhibitors (NRTIs) plus one of either a ritonavir-boosted protease inhibitor, a non-nucleoside reverse transcriptase inhibitor or an integrase inhibitor.

9.4 SEXUALLY TRANSMITTED INFECTIONS

1. Match the condition to the correct organism description.

Condition	Organism
Trichomonas vaginalis	Protozoon
Chlamydia	Gram-negative organism
Syphilis	Spirochaete
Gonorrhoea	Gram-negative diplococci
Genital herpes	Virus

2. Name three complications of untreated chlamydia infection.

   Complications of an untreated chlamydia infection include:

   Women: PID, endometritis, salpingitis, infertility, perihepatitis (Fitz-Hugh–Curtis syndrome), ectopic pregnancy, reactive arthritis.

   Men: epididymo-orchitis, reactive arthritis.

3. What are the management options for a patient with an uncomplicated anogenital gonorrhoea infection?

- Conservative management:
  - Patients should ideally be referred to a GUM clinic for education about the condition and safe sexual practice
  - Patients should be encouraged to engage in patient-led partner notification to encourage them to be tested for STIs and treated for gonorrhoea
  - Patients should be screened for other STIs and advised to abstain from sexual intercourse until they and their partners have completed treatment (or after 7 days following azithromycin treatment)
- Medical management:
  - For a confirmed or suspected uncomplicated anogenital infection, a combination of IM ceftriaxone and oral azithromycin is recommended
  - A test of cure is recommended and follow-up is recommended 2 weeks after treatment to confirm resolution of symptoms/infection, confirm partner notification and reinforce safe sexual practice

4. Describe the stages of an untreated syphilis infection.

Primary syphilis: Usually occurs following an incubation period of approximately 9–90 days. Signs include the development of chancres (often painless genital ulcers) that typically resolve spontaneously.

Secondary syphilis: Approximately 25% of patients with primary syphilis will go on to the secondary stage. Features of secondary syphilis appear 4–10 weeks after the chancres and include:

- Skin manifestations: Widespread mucocutaneous rash
- Lymphadenopathy, commonly inguinal and cervical
- Condylomata lata (wart-like lesions on genitals)
- Neurological manifestations: Meningitis, cranial nerve palsies, optic neuropathy, uveitis
- Systemic manifestations: Hepatitis, glomerulonephritis, splenomegaly

Latent disease: Approximately 3–12 weeks following secondary syphilis, the disease will enter a latent stage where patients are completely asymptomatic. One-quarter of these patients may experience a recurrence of secondary disease. Latent disease is classified into two stages: early latent syphilis – where a person has been infected for less than 2 years, and late latent syphilis where infection has been present for over 2 years.

Tertiary syphilis occurs in approximately one-third of untreated patients 20–40 years after the initial infection. Late disease can manifest in neurological, cardiovascular or gummatous complications.

5. How does a genital ulcer caused by genital herpes differ from an ulcer caused by primary syphilis?

Classically, an ulcer caused by primary syphilis (chancre) is a **painless** ulcer, whereas ulcers caused by genital herpes are classically **painful**.

CHAPTER 10: DERMATOLOGY

10.1 ECZEMA

1. Which surfaces does eczema typically affect?

   Flexor surfaces.

2. What are the treatment options available for a flare of atopic eczema?

   Emollients, topical corticosteroids and antihistamines if there is itch or urticaria.

3. What are the complications of atopic eczema?

   Infection: *Staphylococcus aureus* infection, eczema herpeticum, fungal infections.

   Psychosocial problems: Behavioural problems and depression.

10.2 PSORIASIS

1. What are the nail changes that may be found in psoriasis?

   Pitting, onycholysis, subungual hyperkeratosis.

2. Patients with psoriasis are at increased risk of which conditions?

   Psoriatic arthritis, venous thromboembolism, cardiovascular disease, metabolic syndrome, psoriatic arthritis, depression.

3. What are the medical treatment options for the treatment of psoriasis as recommended by NICE?

   Regular emollient use.

   First line: Topical corticosteroid and vitamin D analogue once daily.

   Second line: Vitamin D analogue twice daily.

   Third line: Potent corticosteroid twice daily for 4 weeks or coal tar preparation once or twice daily.

10.3 SKIN CANCER

1. What is the main risk factor for the development of skin cancer?

   UV ray exposure.

2. What is the main differential diagnosis for a patient presenting with a squamous cell carcinoma?

   Keratocanthoma.

3. What does the ABCDE criteria stand for in the assessment of pigmented lesions?

   Asymmetry of lesion, Border (irregular), Colour (variegated), Diameter >6 mm, Enlargement/Evolution.

4. Is there any known precancerous condition leading to development of a BCC?

   No, BCC develops de novo.

CHAPTER 11: ORTHOPAEDICS

11.1 OSTEOARTHRITIS

1. Name three features on examination that would be suggestive of hip osteoarthritis.

   Any three from:
   - Wasting of gluteal muscles
   - Antalgic gait
   - Apparent shortening of affected leg
   - Painful movement of the hip
   - May have nodes on hands or a joint effusion hip
   - Restricted movement of the hip
   - Crepitus

2. What are the x-ray features of an osteoarthritic joint?

   the x-ray changes in osteoarthritis can be remembered by the mnemonic **LOSS: L**oss of joint space, **O**steophytes, **S**ubchondral cysts, **S**ubchondral sclerosis.

3. What non-pharmacological therapies are available to treat osteoarthritis?

   Non-pharmacological therapies include:
   - Weight loss
   - Exercise
   - Local heat and ice packs
   - Joint supports
   - Physiotherapy
   - Transcutaneous nerve stimulation

4. What pharmacological therapies are available to treat osteoarthritis?

   Pharmacological therapies include:
   - Paracetamol
   - NSAIDs (with co-prescribed proton pump inhibitor)
   - Opioids (such as codeine)
   - Intra-articular joint injection

5. What are the specific complications of a total knee replacement?

   Specific complications of a total knee replacement include:
   - Intraoperative: Tibial fracture
   - Immediate: Vascular injury
   - Early: DVT/PE, peroneal nerve palsy, infection
   - Late: Infection, instability

11.2 HIP FRACTURES

1. Name three risk factors for having a hip fracture.

   Any three from:
   - Increasing age
   - Female sex
   - Osteoporosis
   - Osteomalacia
   - History of falls
   - Fall risk factors (e.g. poor vision, instability, dementia, etc.)

2. What types of hip fracture are there?

   Hip fractures are broadly divided into intracapsular or extracapsular depending on whether they occur within or outside the femoral capsule.

3. What is the Garden classification?

   The Garden classification is a system used to divide intracapsular hip fractures based on the displacement of the fracture and whether it extends the length of the femoral neck.

4. Which investigations should be performed in a patient prior to hip fracture surgery?
   - Pre-surgery investigations include:
   - Bedside tests: Urinalysis, ECG
   - Bloods: FBC, LFTs, calcium, U&Es, clotting, group and save, glucose
   - Imaging: CXR, hip fracture

5. Name three complications of fractures.

   Any three from:
   - Tissue damage (haemorrhage, shock, infection, rhabdomyolysis)
   - Compartment syndrome (increase in pressure within a closed fascial compartment)
   - Neurological damage (e.g. neuropraxia, pain)
   - Avascular necrosis
   - Malunion

CHAPTER 12: GENERAL SURGERY

12.1 GALLSTONES

1. What is the most common type of gallstone?

   Cholesterol gallstones are the most common type of gallstone.

2. Name three ways in which gallstones can present.

   Gallstones may be asymptomatic but may present as biliary colic, acute cholecystitis, acute pancreatitis, ascending cholangitis, a mucocele or a gallstone ileus.

3. What are the complications of a cholecystectomy?

   Complications of a cholecystectomy can be divided into general and specific complications. Specific complications of this surgery include damage to local structures such as the cystic or hepatic artery (resulting in haemorrhage), bile leakage, bile duct injury, intestine damage or postcholecystectomy syndrome.

12.2 PANCREATITIS

1. What are the causes of pancreatitis?

   Causes of pancreatitis can be remembered by the mnemonic **GET SMASH³ED**: **G**allstones (most common cause in women), **E**thanol (most common cause in men), **T**rauma, **S**teroids, **M**umps (other viruses include Coxsackie B/Epstein–Barr), **A**utoimmune (e.g. polyarteritis nodosa/SLE), **S**corpion venom and snake bites, **H**ypertriglyceridaemia, **H**ypercalcaemia, **H**ypothermia, **E**RCP, **D**rugs (azathioprine, bendroflumethiazide, furosemide, steroids, sodium valproate).

2. What scoring systems can be used to grade the severity of acute pancreatitis?

   Scoring systems used in pancreatitis include the Glasgow score, the Ranson score and the APACHE score.

3. What are the complications of pancreatitis?

   The complications of pancreatitis can be divided into early and late.

   Early complications include shock and renal failure, acute respiratory distress syndrome, hypocalcaemia and hyperglycaemia. Late complications include pancreatic pseudocyst formation, pancreatic necrosis, type 1 diabetes mellitus and chronic pancreatitis.

12.3 HERNIAS AND GROIN LUMPS

1. What is the difference aetiologically between indirect and direct inguinal hernias?

   Indirect inguinal hernias may occur due to a patent processus vaginalis through the deep inguinal ring. Direct inguinal hernias occur due to a weakness or defect in the abdominal wall.

2. What are the borders and significance of Hesselbach's triangle?

   Hesselbach's triangle is formed from the inferior epigastric vessels, the rectus sheath and the inguinal ligament. It is significant because direct inguinal hernias originate within Hesselbach's triangle, whereas indirect inguinal hernias originate lateral to Hesselbach's triangle at the deep inguinal ring.

3. What are the complications of inguinal hernia repair surgery?

   Complications of inguinal hernia repair surgery can be divided into general and specific complications. Specific complications of this surgery include damage to local structures such as the ilioinguinal nerve, resulting in pain/paraesthesia, the vas deferens or the blood supply to the testicle.

12.4 BREAST CANCER

1. Name three risk factors for developing breast cancer.

   Any three from: Family history, BRCA1/2 mutations, ↑ oestrogen exposure (nulliparity, first pregnancy > age 30, early menarche, late menopause, HRT, COCP use, obesity), previous breast cancer, ↑ age and never breastfeeding.

2. What is involved in a triple assessment in a patient with a breast lump?

   A triple assessment for a breast lump involves:
   - Clinical examination
   - Imaging: USS (if <35) or mammography (if >35)
   - Pathological analysis: Fine-needle aspiration or tissue biopsy

3. What are the treatment options for a patient with breast cancer?

   Depending on the stage of the breast cancer options include surgery, hormone therapies, biological therapy, chemotherapy and radiotherapy. For Stage 1 and 2 breast cancers, surgery is indicated with hormone and biological adjuvant therapy (if receptor positive). For Stage 3 and 4, chemotherapy and palliation with adjuvant hormone and biological therapy is indicated.

12.5 COLORECTAL CANCER

1. How do right-sided and left-sided colorectal carcinomas classically present?

   Classically, right-sided cancers present with weight loss and iron deficiency anaemia. Left-sided cancers present with altered bowel habit, PR bleeding, tenesmus or large bowel obstruction.

2. What are the risk factors for the development of colorectal carcinoma?

   Risk factors for the development of colorectal carcinoma include neoplastic polyps, inflammatory bowel disease (UC > CD), low-fibre diet, smoking, previous cancer and familial cancer syndromes.

3. What are the complications of a stoma?

   Stoma complications include fluid loss (from high-output stoma), bowel obstruction, parastomal hernia, odour, skin irritation and psychological complications.

CHAPTER 13: UROLOGY

13.1 RENAL/URETERIC STONES

1. Which is the most common type of renal stone by composition?

   Calcium type stones – often a combination of calcium oxalate and calcium phosphate.

2. Where are the three locations where renal stones usually obstruct?

   The pelvi-ureteric junction (PUJ), the mid-ureter where the ureter crosses the iliac vessels and the vesico-ureteric junction (VUJ).

3. What management options are available for renal stones <5 mm without evidence of obstruction or anatomical abnormality?

   Non-pharmacological management (wait until the stone passes).

   Pharmacological expulsion therapy (using an alpha-blocker, e.g. tamsulosin).

13.2 BENIGN PROSTATIC ENLARGEMENT AND LOWER URINARY TRACT SYMPTOMS

1. Name three voiding and three storage lower urinary tract symptoms that patients with BPE may present with.

   Any three from each:

   - Voiding: Poor stream, double voiding, hesitancy, terminal dribbling, straining to void and feeling of incomplete emptying.
   - Storage: Increased frequency, nocturia, urgency and dysuria.

2. Describe the pharmacological treatment options for BPE and their mechanism of action.

   Alpha-blockers (e.g. tamsulosin): Work by relaxing prostate smooth muscle.

   5-alpha-reductase inhibitors (e.g. finasteride): Inhibit conversion of testosterone to dihydrotestosterone and cause shrinkage of the prostate.

   Antimuscarinics (e.g. tolterodine): Block the action of acetylcholine binding on muscarinic receptors in the bladder smooth muscle to inhibit their contraction.

3. What surgical options are there for managing BPH?

   Surgical options include:

   - Transurethral resection of the prostate (TURP)
   - Transurethral vaporisation of the prostate (TUVP)
   - Transurethral laser enucleation of the prostate
   - Open prostatectomy

13.3 PROSTATE CANCER

1. Prostate cancers are adenocarcinomas that generally affect which part of the prostate gland?

   The majority of adenocarcinomas affect the **outer zone** of prostate gland. This is why urinary symptoms are a later sign of prostate cancer as the prostatic urethra is located in the inner or transitional zone.

2. What are the causes for a raised PSA?

   Causes of a raised PSA include:

   - Prostate cancer
   - Benign prostatic hypertrophy
   - Prostatitis
   - UTI
   - Ejaculation
   - Recent vigorous exercise

3. Describe the three main stages of prostate cancer and possible treatment options for them.

   Prostate cancers are primarily classified by their stage as localised, locally advanced or metastatic. Within the localised prostate cancer group, these can be further risk stratified by their clinical stage, Gleason or ISUP.

   Localised disease: Active surveillance/watchful waiting, radical prostatectomy, brachytherapy or external beam radiotherapy depending on the risk stratification.

   Locally advanced disease: Usually external beam radiotherapy with androgen deprivation therapy and occasionally radical prostatectomy in selected cases.

   Metastatic disease: Palliative androgen deprivation therapy (e.g. goserelin) potentially with chemotherapy (e.g. docetaxel) or specialist androgen blockade (e.g. abiraterone).

CHAPTER 14: VASCULAR SURGERY

14.1 PERIPHERAL ARTERIAL DISEASE

1. What are the risk factors for developing peripheral arterial disease?

   The risk factors for peripheral arterial disease can be divided into modifiable and non-modifiable.

   Modifiable risk factors include hypertension, **smoking**, ↑ cholesterol, diabetes, obesity, sedentary lifestyle.

   Non-modifiable risk factors include family history, increasing age, sex (M > F until menopause, when M = F).

2. What are the presenting features of an acute ischaemic limb?

   The presenting features of an acute ischaemic limb can be remembered by the **6 P**s: **P**ain, **P**allor, **P**araesthesia, **P**aralysis, **P**erishingly cold, **P**ulselessness.

3. What management options are available for treating peripheral arterial disease?

   Management options for peripheral arterial disease include non-pharmacological measures (education about the condition, manage lifestyle factors [e.g. stop smoking] and a supervised exercise regime). Pharmacological management includes managing cardiovascular risk (secondary prevention medications) and symptomatic treatment (e.g. naftidrofuryl oxalate). Surgical treatments include angioplasty and bypass surgery.

14.2 VENOUS INSUFFICIENCY

1. What are the complications of varicose veins?

   Complications of varicose veins include haemorrhage, varicose eczema, venous ulceration, thrombophlebitis, oedema, lipodermatosclerosis and haemosiderin deposition.

2. What are the surgical options for treating varicose veins?

   Surgical treatment options include removal, ligation, foam sclerotherapy and endothermal ablation.

3. Name three risk factors for the development of a deep vein thrombosis.

   Any three from: Previous DVT, malignancy, increasing age, obesity, heart failure, thrombophilia, vascular wall trauma (e.g. vasculitis), immobility, hormone treatment (e.g. HRT), pregnancy, dehydration and recent surgery.

4. What are the treatment options for an unprovoked DVT?

   Patients should initially be treated with a LMWH or fondaparinux. Following this, warfarin or an NOAC should be started and continued for up to 6 months for unprovoked DVTs.

14.3 ABDOMINAL AORTIC ANEURYSM

1. Where do the majority of abdominal aortic aneurysms occur?

   Ninety percent of AAAs occur below the renal arteries.

2. At what aneurysm size are patients referred to vascular surgery following screening?

   When the abdominal aortic aneurysm is or exceeds 5.5 cm in diameter.

3. What non-pharmacological management options are recommended for patients with an abdominal aortic aneurysm?

   Non-pharmacological management options include lifestyle changes (e.g. stop smoking, regular exercise, losing weight, healthy eating) and managing cardiovascular risk with secondary prevention medications.

CHAPTER 15: EAR, NOSE AND THROAT

15.1 VERTIGO

1. What is the most commonly diagnosed cause of vertigo?

   Benign paroxysmal positional vertigo (BPPV).

2. What is the difference between acute vestibular neuronitis and acute labyrinthitis?

   In acute vestibular neuronitis there is only inflammation of the vestibular nerve, so there is vertigo without hearing loss. In acute labyrinthitis there is inflammation of the entire labyrinth, so patients experience vertigo with hearing loss.

3. What investigation needs to be performed before the diagnosis of Menière's disease and why?

   MRI: To exclude an acoustic neuroma.

4. A 76-year-old woman is diagnosed with Menière's disease. What treatment options are available to her?

   Non-pharmacological options include sound therapy and relaxation techniques. Pharmacological options include prochlorperazine or an antihistamine. Betahistine can be used to prevent attacks. Surgical options include injected intratympanic ototoxic drugs directly into the middle ear.

5. What treatment options are available for symptomatic relief of acute vestibular neuronitis and labyrinthitis?

   Cyclizine or prochlorperazine can be used to relieve nausea, vomiting and vertigo in acute vestibular neuronitis and acute labyrinthitis.

15.2 HEARING LOSS

1. Classify the following causes of hearing loss by whether they predominantly cause:

   a. Conductive hearing loss

   b. Sensorineural hearing loss
      i. Acoustic neuroma – **b**
      ii. Otosclerosis – **a**
      iii. Wax – **a**
      iv. Presbyacusis – **b**
      v. Ramsay–Hunt syndrome – **b**
      vi. Noise-induced hearing loss – **b**
      vii. Otitis media – **a**
      viii. Menière's disease – **b**

2. What red flag features should you look for when a patient presents with acute otitis media?

   Meningitis, mastoiditis or facial nerve paralysis.

3. In which scenarios when a patient presents with hearing loss should you always refer to ENT?
   - Conductive deafness of unknown cause
   - Sudden deafness if no wax is visible on examination
   - Asymmetrical deafness

4. Which medications can lead to a sensorineural hearing loss?
   - Loop diuretics
   - Aminoglycosides

INDEX